THE MACRO DIET COOKBOOK FOR BEGINNERS
2024

A Comprehensive Guide to Achieving Your
Health and Fitness Goals.

VIVIAN I. DAVID

Copyright © 2024 [VIVIAN I. DAVID]

TABLE OF CONTENTS

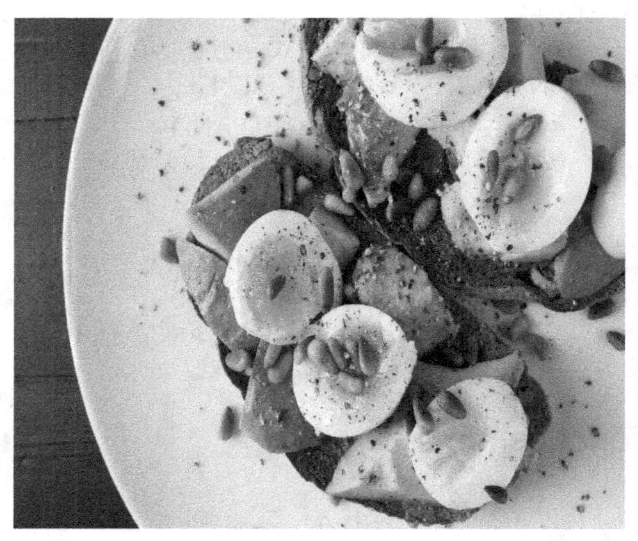

INTRODUCTION

Once upon a time, in a small town nestled amidst rolling green hills, there lived a woman named Rene. Rene had always been passionate about living a healthy and vibrant life, but she found herself trapped in a cycle of yo-yo dieting and frustration. She longed for a sustainable approach to nourishing her body and achieving her health and fitness goals.

One sunny morning, as Rene sat at her kitchen table sipping her coffee, a package arrived at her doorstep. Intrigued, she opened it to find a beautifully bound book, titled "The Macro Diet Cookbook for Beginners 2024: A Comprehensive Guide to Achieving Your Health and Fitness Goals." A surge of excitement coursed through Rene's veins as she realized that this book held the key to her long-awaited transformation.

Curiosity piqued, Rene settled into her favorite armchair, flipping open the book's pages. As she delved into the introduction, she discovered a captivating story, one that would forever change her perspective on food and ignite her determination to reclaim her health.

The story began with a young woman named Crystal, who, like Rene, had struggled for years to find a sustainable path to a healthier lifestyle. Crystal's days were filled with fatigue, self-doubt, and a constant battle with her weight. She had tried countless diets and exercise routines, but none seemed to bring her the lasting results she craved. One fateful day, during a routine visit to her doctor, Crystal was introduced to the concept of the macro diet. Intrigued, she embarked on a journey of discovery, immersing herself in books, scientific studies, and personal testimonies. As she delved deeper, Crystal realized that the macro diet was not just another restrictive plan but a flexible and empowering way to nourish her body.

Determined to transform her life, Crystal embraced the macro diet with unwavering commitment. She learned to calculate her macronutrient needs, finding the perfect balance of carbohydrates, proteins, and fats to fuel her body and support her goals. With each passing day, Crystal's energy levels soared, her body transformed, and her self-confidence grew.
But it wasn't just the physical changes that captivated Crystal. The macro diet opened her eyes to a world of vibrant flavors and culinary creativity. She discovered a plethora of delicious recipes that not only satisfied her taste buds but also nourished her body from within.

Crystal's journey inspired her to share her newfound knowledge and recipes with others who, like her, had longed for a sustainable approach to health. She poured her heart and soul into creating "The Macro Diet Cookbook for Beginners 2024," a comprehensive guide that would empower individuals to achieve their health and fitness goals. The cookbook was a treasure trove of recipes, practical tips, and motivational stories. From mouthwatering breakfast bowls and satisfying lunches to hearty dinners and guilt-free desserts, Crystal had meticulously crafted a collection of dishes that would delight the taste buds while keeping macros in check.

As Rene immersed herself in the pages of the cookbook, she felt a renewed sense of hope and determination. She realized that the journey towards health and fitness wasn't about deprivation or punishment; it was about nourishing her body, embracing balance, and finding joy in the process.

With the cookbook as her guide, Rene embarked on her own macro diet adventure. She learned to love the process of planning and preparing meals, relishing in the knowledge that each dish was a step towards her goals. She discovered new flavors, experimented with ingredients, and shared her culinary delights with friends and family, who were amazed by her newfound vitality and zest for life.

Through her commitment and dedication, Rene transformed not only her physical health but also her mindset. She learned to appreciate her body for all the incredible things it could do and celebrated each small victory along the way.

As Rene closed the book, she felt a surge of excitement and possibility. She knew that her journey towards health and fitness would have its challenges, but armed with the knowledge, inspiration, and delicious recipes from "The Macro Diet Cookbook for Beginners 2024," she was ready to conquer them all.
And so, Rene set forth on her path, fueled by the stories of Crystal and countless others who had embraced the macro diet and achieved their health and fitness goals. With every meal she prepared, every milestone she reached, and every obstacle she overcame, Rene became a living testament to the transformative power of the macro diet.

As you embark on your own journey towards health and vitality, remember Rene's story, and let it be a beacon of hope and inspiration. With "The Macro Diet Cookbook for Beginners 2024" as your guide, you too can achieve your health and fitness goals, one delicious and macro-friendly meal at a time.

CHAPTER 1:

UNDERSTANDING THE MACRO DIET

-WHAT IS THE MACRO DIET?

The term "macro diet" refers to a dietary approach that focuses on macronutrients, which are the three essential components of our diet: carbohydrates, proteins, and fats. The concept behind the macro diet is to carefully balance and track the intake of these macronutrients to achieve specific health or fitness goals.

The macro diet gained popularity because it emphasizes the importance of understanding the composition of food and how it affects our bodies. By tracking and manipulating macronutrient ratios, individuals can customize their diet to support weight loss, muscle gain, athletic performance, or overall well-being.

Numerous renowned authors and experts have provided valuable insights into the meaning of the macro diet. Let's explore a few of their definitions:

1. Lyle McDonald: Lyle McDonald, a prominent author and nutrition specialist, explains the macro diet in his book "The Ketogenic Diet." He defines it as a method of eating that involves monitoring and adjusting

macronutrient intake to achieve desired body composition goals.

2. Layne Norton: Dr. Layne Norton, a renowned physique coach and researcher, discusses the macro diet in his works. He describes it as a flexible approach that allows individuals to manipulate their macronutrient intake to meet their specific needs and preferences while maintaining overall calorie balance.

3. Precision Nutrition: The team at Precision Nutrition, a leading authority in nutrition coaching, defines the macro diet as a way of eating that focuses on consuming the right amounts of carbohydrates, proteins, and fats to support individual goals. They emphasize the importance of balance and personalization.

It's important to note that the macro diet is not a one-size-fits-all approach. The specific macronutrient ratios and overall calorie intake can vary based on individual goals, such as weight loss, muscle gain, or athletic performance. Consulting with a registered dietitian or nutritionist can provide personalized guidance and help ensure that the macro diet aligns with your specific needs and health considerations.

Remember, while the macro diet can be a helpful tool for managing body composition and overall well-being, it's always essential to prioritize the quality of the food sources within each macronutrient category. Opting for whole, unprocessed foods and considering factors like micronutrient content, fiber, and overall dietary diversity can contribute to long-term health benefits.

-BENEFITS OF THE MACRO DIET

The macro diet, also known as flexible dieting or IIFYM (If It Fits Your Macros), can offer several benefits:

1. Flexible Food Choices: The macro diet focuses on tracking and balancing macronutrients—carbohydrates, proteins, and fats—rather than specific foods. This flexibility allows you to enjoy a wide variety of foods while still meeting your nutritional goals.

2. Personalized Approach: The macro diet can be tailored to your individual needs and preferences. By calculating your specific macronutrient targets based on your goals (such as weight loss, muscle gain, or maintenance), you can create a plan that suits your unique requirements.

3. Sustainable Weight Management: Since the macro diet does not restrict specific food groups, it can be easier to stick to long-term. This can promote sustainable weight management as it focuses on overall calorie control and meeting nutrient needs while allowing for occasional indulgences.

4. Increased Awareness: Tracking macronutrients can enhance your awareness of portion sizes, food

composition, and the overall nutritional value of what you eat. This can help you make more informed choices and develop a healthier relationship with food.

5. Support for Fitness Goals: The macro diet can be beneficial for individuals involved in fitness or strength training. By adjusting macronutrient ratios and overall calorie intake, it allows for optimized fueling and muscle recovery.

6. Improved Body Composition: By tracking macronutrients and maintaining a calorie deficit or surplus as needed, the macro diet can help you achieve and maintain a healthier body composition, such as reducing body fat while preserving lean muscle mass.

It's important to note that while the macro diet offers flexibility, it's still essential to prioritize nutrient-dense foods, such as fruits, vegetables, lean proteins, and healthy fats, to meet your micronutrient needs and support overall health. Consulting a registered dietitian or nutritionist can provide personalized guidance on implementing the macro diet effectively.

-HOW TO CALCULATE YOUR MACROS AND SETTING REALISTIC GOALS

Calculating your macros and setting realistic goals are important steps in achieving a balanced and sustainable approach to nutrition and fitness. Let's break down each topic:

1. CALCULATING YOUR MACROS:

Macros, short for macronutrients, refer to the three main nutrients that provide energy to your body: carbohydrates, proteins, and fats. Determining your macro intake involves establishing the optimal ratio of these nutrients based on your goals and lifestyle. Here's a step-by-step guide:

a. Define Your Goal: Determine whether you want to lose weight, gain muscle, or maintain your current weight. Each goal has different macro requirements.

b. Calculate Your Total Daily Energy Expenditure (TDEE): TDEE represents the total number of calories your body needs to maintain its current weight. Use an online calculator that takes into account your age, gender, weight, height, and activity level.

c. Set Caloric Intake: Based on your goal, adjust your caloric intake. Create a calorie deficit by consuming fewer calories than TDEE in other to lose weight. To gain weight, create a calorie surplus by consuming more calories.

d. Determine Macro Ratios: Generally, a common starting point is to allocate 45-65% of calories to carbohydrates, 20-35% to fats, and 10-35% to proteins.

e. Calculate Macros: Convert your macronutrient ratios into grams. Multiply your total daily calorie intake by the percentage allocated to each macro. For example, if your target calorie intake is 2000 calories and you want 30% of your calories to come from protein, you would multiply 2000 by 0.30 to get 600 calories from protein. Since protein contains 4 calories per gram, divide 600 by 4 to get 150 grams of protein.

Therefore, always remember that these ratios are starting points, and you may need to adjust them based on personal preferences, dietary restrictions, and how your body responds to different ratios.

2. SETTING REALISTIC GOALS:
Setting realistic goals is crucial for long-term success. Here are some tips to help you set achievable objectives:

a. Be Specific: Clearly define your goals, whether it's losing a certain amount of weight, increasing muscle mass, or improving athletic performance. The more specific your goal, the easier it is to measure progress.

b. Set Measurable Targets: Break your larger goal into smaller, manageable milestones. For instance, if your goal is to lose 20 pounds, set smaller targets of 2-3 pounds per month.

c. Make It Time-Bound: Assign a timeframe to your goals. This adds urgency and accountability. Be realistic with the timeline, considering factors such as your starting point, lifestyle, and any potential obstacles.

d. Consider Your Lifestyle: Ensure your goals align with your lifestyle and are sustainable in the long run. If you set goals that require drastic changes or aren't compatible with your daily routine, it can be challenging to maintain motivation.

e. Celebrate Progress: Acknowledge and celebrate your accomplishments along the way. This helps maintain motivation and reinforces positive behavior.

f. Seek Professional Guidance: Consulting with a registered dietitian or a fitness professional can provide personalized guidance and help you set realistic goals based on your unique circumstances.

Moreover, bear it in mind that progress takes time, and it's important to focus on sustainable changes rather than quick fixes. Pay attention to your body, be patient, and make adjustments if the need be.

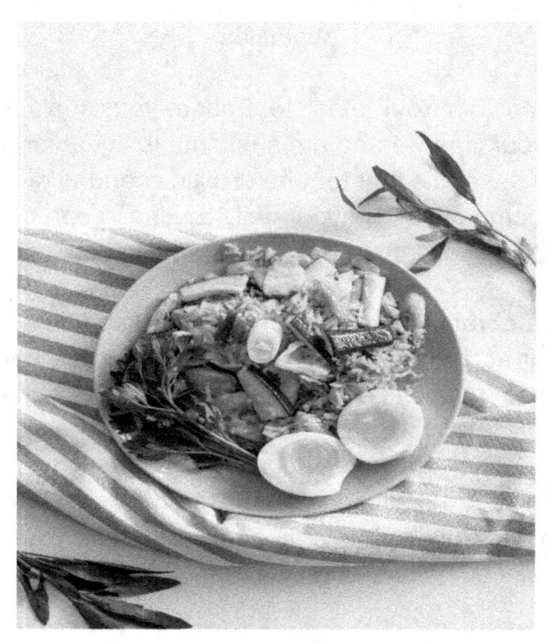

CHAPTER 2:

BUILDING A BALANCED PLATE

-MACRONUTRIENTS: PROTEIN, CARBOHYDRATES, AND FATS.

Macros, short for macronutrients, are the three main categories of nutrients that our bodies require in large quantities to function properly: carbohydrates, proteins, and fats. Understanding these macros is crucial for maintaining a healthy and balanced diet. Let's delve into each one and explore their roles and significance.

1. CARBOHYDRATES:

Carbohydrates are the body's primary source of energy. They include carbon, hydrogen, and oxygen atoms. Common sources of carbohydrates include grains, fruits, vegetables, legumes, and dairy products. Carbohydrates are classified into three main types: sugars, starches, and dietary fiber.

- Sugars: These are simple carbohydrates found in foods like table sugar, honey, and fruits. They provide a rapid energy boost and digest quickly. However, excessive sugar consumption can lead to health issues like weight gain and an increased risk of diabetes.

- Starches: These complex carbohydrates are present in foods like potatoes, rice, bread, and pasta. Starches take longer to digest, providing sustained energy levels. Whole grains are a healthier choice because they contain more fiber and nutrients than refined grains.

- Dietary Fiber: Fiber, found in fruits, vegetables, whole grains, and legumes, is a type of carbohydrate that cannot be digested by the body. It aids in digestion, promotes bowel regularity, and helps control blood sugar levels. High-fiber foods are beneficial for weight management and reducing the risk of heart disease.

2. PROTEINS:

The synthesis, maintenance, and repair of bodily tissues depend on proteins. Amino acids, the building blocks of proteins, make up their composition. Dairy products, beans, eggs, fish, poultry, and meat are examples of foods high in protein.. the following are some key points about proteins:

- Amino Acids: There are 20 different amino acids, nine of which are essential, meaning our bodies cannot produce them and must obtain them through diet. Animal-based proteins generally provide all essential amino acids, while plant-based proteins may require combining different sources to ensure adequate intake.

- Muscle Development: Proteins play a crucial role in muscle growth and repair. Athletes, bodybuilders, and individuals engaging in regular exercise often require higher protein intake to support muscle development and recovery.

- Satiety and Weight Management: Protein-rich foods tend to be more satisfying and can help control appetite. They have a higher thermic effect, meaning the body expends more energy to digest and process them. Including protein in meals can contribute to weight management efforts.

3. FATS:
Fats are a concentrated source of energy, providing more than double the calories per gram compared to carbohydrates and proteins. While fats have traditionally received a negative reputation, it's important to understand that they are essential for various bodily functions. Here are the key aspects of fats:

- Types of Fats: There are different types of fats, including saturated fats, trans fats, monounsaturated fats, and polyunsaturated fats. Saturated and trans fats, commonly found in high-fat animal products and processed foods, should be limited due to their association with cardiovascular diseases. Monounsaturated and polyunsaturated fats, found in foods like avocados, nuts, seeds, and fatty fish, are considered healthier options.

- Nutrient Absorption: Fats aid in the absorption of fat-soluble vitamins (A, D, E, and K) and other fat-soluble compounds. Including small amounts of healthy fats in meals can enhance the absorption of these nutrients.

- Hormone Production: Fats are involved in the production of hormones and help regulate various bodily processes. It also provides insulation and protection for organs.

While understanding macros is important, it's essential to recognize that a healthy diet is about balance and moderation. The optimal macro ratio varies depending on factors such as age, sex, activity level, and overall health goals. However, Consulting with a registered dietitian or nutritionist can provide personalized guidance to meet individual needs and maintain a well-rounded diet.

-THE IMPORTANCE OF PORTION CONTROL

Portion control is a fundamental aspect of the macro diet, and its importance cannot be overstated. The macro diet, also known as flexible dieting or counting macros, focuses on tracking and balancing macronutrients—carbohydrates, proteins, and fats—to achieve specific health and fitness goals. While macronutrient ratios are essential, the quantity of food consumed plays a crucial role in achieving desired results, and that is where portion control comes into play.

One of the primary benefits of portion control in the macro diet is calorie management. By controlling portion sizes, individuals can effectively manage their caloric intake. This is critical because weight loss or gain is ultimately determined by the energy balance equation, which states that weight is influenced by the number of calories consumed versus the number of calories expended. Consuming larger portions can lead to an excess of calories, potentially hindering weight loss goals or causing weight gain. Conversely, consuming smaller portions can create a calorie deficit, leading to weight loss.

Another advantage of portion control is maintaining a balanced macronutrient intake. While tracking macros allows for flexibility in food choices, portion control ensures that the desired macronutrient ratios are met. For example, if a person's goal is to consume 40% of calories from carbohydrates, 30% from protein, and 30% from fat, portion control helps in achieving these ratios by regulating the amount of each macronutrient consumed. By adhering to portion sizes, individuals can design meals that align with their specific macro goals, supporting their overall health and fitness objectives.

Portion control also promotes mindful eating. In today's fast-paced world, it's easy to lose track of how much we consume. Oversized portions have become the norm, leading to overeating and potential weight gain. By practicing portion control, individuals become more aware of their serving sizes and develop a better understanding of their body's needs. They become more in tune with hunger and satiety cues, allowing them to eat in moderation and avoid overindulging. This mindfulness fosters a healthier relationship with food and enhances overall dietary success.

Furthermore, portion control helps in preventing or managing chronic conditions such as obesity, diabetes, and cardiovascular diseases. Overeating and consuming excessively large portions can contribute to weight gain and exacerbate health issues. By controlling portion sizes, individuals can regulate their calorie intake and maintain a healthy weight. Additionally, portion control assists in managing blood sugar levels, as it helps individuals consume an appropriate amount of carbohydrates while balancing them with protein and fat. This can be beneficial for those with diabetes or insulin resistance.

In conclusion, portion control plays a vital role in the macro diet. It facilitates calorie management, supports balanced macronutrient intake, encourages mindful eating, and aids in the prevention and management of chronic conditions. By practicing portion control, individuals can optimize their nutrition, achieve their health and fitness goals, and cultivate a sustainable and balanced approach to eating. Remember, it's not just about what you eat but also how much you eat that matters when it comes to the macro diet.

-CHOOSING HIGH-QUALITY INGREDIENTS

When following a macro diet, it's important to choose high-quality ingredients to meet your nutritional needs. Here are some tips for selecting quality ingredients:

1. Lean Proteins: Opt for lean sources of protein like skinless chicken breast, turkey, fish, tofu, or legumes. Look for organic, grass-fed, or wild-caught options when possible.

2. Whole Grains: Choose whole grains like quinoa, brown rice, whole wheat bread, or oats. These provide fiber, vitamins, and minerals. Avoid refined grains.

3. **Healthy Fats:** Its sources include avocados, nuts, seeds, and olive oil. These offer essential fatty acids and help you feel satisfied.

4. Fresh Fruits and Vegetables: Incorporate a variety of colorful fruits and vegetables into your diet to ensure a wide range of nutrients. Aim for organic produce when feasible.

5. Minimize Processed Foods: Limit processed foods, as they often contain additives, preservatives, and unhealthy trans fats. Instead, focus on whole, unprocessed foods.

6. Read Labels: Check nutrition labels for information on ingredients, serving sizes, and macronutrient content. Look for minimal additives and avoid high sugar or sodium content.

Remember, the goal of a macro diet is to balance your macronutrient intake. By choosing high-quality ingredients, you can optimize your nutrition and support your overall health.

-INCORPORATING FRUITS AND VEGETABLES

Incorporating fruits and vegetables into a macro diet is essential for maximizing nutrition while maintaining the desired macronutrient balance. Here are some extensive tips on how to do so effectively:

1. Plan Ahead: Plan your meals and snacks in advance to ensure that you have a variety of fruits and vegetables included in your daily intake. This will help you meet your macronutrient goals while also getting the necessary vitamins, minerals, and fiber from plant-based foods.

2. Balance Macronutrients: When incorporating fruits and vegetables into a macro diet, pay attention to their macronutrient content. While fruits are generally higher in carbohydrates, vegetables tend to be lower in calories and carbohydrates. Consider the macronutrient composition of your other meals and adjust the portion sizes of fruits and vegetables accordingly to maintain the desired balance.

3. Prioritize Non-Starchy Vegetables: Non-starchy vegetables are low in calories and carbohydrates while being rich in fiber and essential nutrients. Examples include leafy greens (spinach, kale, lettuce), cruciferous vegetables (broccoli, cauliflower, Brussels sprouts), peppers, cucumbers, zucchini, and asparagus. These can be consumed in larger quantities without significantly impacting your macronutrient ratios.

4. Choose Lower-Sugar Fruits: While fruits are nutritious and provide essential vitamins and minerals, some are higher in natural sugars than others. Opt for fruits that are lower in sugar, such as berries (strawberries, blueberries, raspberries), citrus fruits (grapefruits, oranges), and melons (watermelon, cantaloupe). These can be enjoyed in moderation without spiking blood sugar levels.

5. Incorporate Fruits and Vegetables into Protein Sources: Use fruits and vegetables as accompaniments or additions to your protein sources. For example, pair grilled chicken or fish with a side of steamed broccoli or roasted Brussels sprouts. Top your salads with sliced fruits like strawberries or diced vegetables like cucumbers for added flavor and texture.

6. Smoothie Boost: Include fruits and vegetables in your smoothies to enhance their nutritional value. Blend leafy greens like spinach or kale with low-sugar fruits, such as berries or a small portion of banana. You can also add vegetables like cucumber or celery to boost hydration and fiber content. Be mindful of portion sizes and the overall macronutrient balance in your smoothies.

7. Snack Smartly: Use fruits and vegetables as healthy snacks to satisfy cravings while sticking to your macro goals. Snack on carrot sticks, cherry tomatoes, celery with nut butter, or sliced bell peppers with hummus. Choose fruits like apple slices, pear wedges, or grapes for a naturally sweet and refreshing snack.

8. Get Creative with Recipes: Explore recipes that incorporate fruits and vegetables in innovative ways. For example, make zucchini noodles or cauliflower rice as a low-carb alternative to traditional pasta or rice. Prepare vegetable-based soups or stews and add fruits to salads or stir-fries for added flavor and nutrition.

9. Experiment with Seasonings and Spices: Use herbs, spices, and healthy seasonings to enhance the flavors of your fruits and vegetables. This can make them more enjoyable and help you stick to your macro diet.

10. Embrace Colorful Meals: Aim for a variety of colors on your plate by including a diverse range of fruits and vegetables. Different colors indicate various nutrients and antioxidants, so incorporating a rainbow of produce ensures you're getting a wide range of nutrients.

Remember, the key to incorporating fruits and vegetables into a macro diet is to strike a balance between macronutrient goals and the nutrient density of plant-based foods. By being mindful of portion sizes, choosing lower-sugar options, and getting creative with recipes, you can successfully integrate fruits and vegetables into your macro diet while optimizing your overall nutrition.

-HYDRATION AND ITS ROLE IN THE MACRO DIET

Hydration plays a crucial role in supporting overall health and optimizing the effectiveness of a macro diet. Here's an extensive look at the importance of hydration within a macro diet:

1. Optimal Nutrient Absorption: Staying well-hydrated aids in the absorption and transportation of nutrients throughout the body. Adequate hydration supports the efficient breakdown and digestion of macronutrients (carbohydrates, proteins, and fats), allowing the body to extract essential nutrients and deliver them to cells for energy production and tissue repair.

2. Metabolism and Weight Management: Proper hydration is linked to a healthy metabolism. Studies have shown that adequate hydration can enhance metabolic rate, which may contribute to weight management efforts. It can help optimize the body's ability to utilize macronutrients effectively, supporting energy balance and potentially aiding in weight loss or maintenance.

3. Appetite and Satiety: Sometimes, thirst can be mistaken for hunger. Staying hydrated can help differentiate between hunger and thirst cues, preventing unnecessary snacking or overeating. Drinking water or other hydrating beverages before meals can promote a feeling of fullness, helping to control portion sizes and support adherence to macro diet goals.

4. Digestive Health: Sufficient hydration is essential for maintaining proper digestive function. Water helps soften and move food through the digestive tract, promoting regular bowel movements and preventing constipation. This is especially important when following a macro diet that emphasizes adequate fiber intake from fruits, vegetables, and whole grains.

5. Exercise Performance: Hydration is crucial for exercise performance and recovery. During physical activity, the body loses fluids through sweat, leading to dehydration if not properly replenished. Dehydration can negatively impact performance, energy levels, and recovery. Maintaining hydration levels ensures optimal muscle function, endurance, and nutrient delivery during workouts.

6. Electrolyte Balance: In addition to water, electrolytes like sodium, potassium, magnesium, and calcium are essential for maintaining proper hydration and supporting cellular function. Electrolytes help regulate fluid balance, nerve impulses, muscle contractions, and pH levels in the body. Consuming electrolyte-rich foods or beverages, such as fruits, vegetables, and sports drinks, can aid in replenishing electrolytes lost through sweat.

7. Temperature Regulation: Proper hydration is vital for maintaining a stable body temperature. Water helps dissipate heat through sweat, enabling the body to cool down during physical activity or in hot environments. This is especially important for individuals on a macro diet who may engage in regular exercise or live in warmer climates.

8. Cognitive Function: Dehydration can impair cognitive function, leading to decreased focus, concentration, and mental performance. Staying well-hydrated supports optimal brain function, memory, and overall mental clarity. This is beneficial when following a macro diet that requires attention to macronutrient ratios and portion control.

To ensure adequate hydration while following a macro diet, consider the following tips:

- Drink water regularly throughout the day, aiming for at least 8 cups (64 ounces) or more, depending on individual needs and activity levels.
- Check urine color as a general indicator of hydration. Pale yellow or clear urine usually indicates adequate hydration, while darker urine may suggest the need to increase fluid intake.

- Include hydrating foods in your diet, such as water-rich fruits and vegetables like watermelon, cucumbers, strawberries, and leafy greens.
- Avoid excessive caffeine and alcohol consumption, as they can contribute to dehydration.
- Consider sports drinks or electrolyte-enhanced beverages during intense workouts or prolonged physical activity to replenish electrolytes lost through sweat.
- Stay mindful of hydration during warmer weather, when traveling, or when engaging in activities that promote sweating.

Hence, individual hydration needs may vary based on factors such as age, weight, activity level, and climate. It's important to listen to your body's thirst cues and prioritize regular hydration to support optimal health and the success of your macro diet.

CHAPTER 3:

ESSENTIAL KITCHEN TOOLS AND PANTRY STAPLES

-MUST-HAVE KITCHEN TOOLS FOR MEAL PREPARATION

When following a macro diet, which focuses on consuming specific ratios of macronutrients (carbohydrates, proteins, and fats), having the right kitchen tools can make meal preparation easier and more efficient. These tools can help you accurately measure and portion your ingredients, as well as prepare meals that align with your macro goals. Here are some must-have kitchen tools for meal preparation on a macro diet:

1. Food Scale: A food scale is essential for accurately weighing and portioning ingredients. Measuring food by weight ensures precise tracking of your macronutrient intake.

2. Measuring Cups and Spoons: Measuring cups and spoons are useful for portioning ingredients like grains, liquids, and condiments according to your macros. Opt for a set with clear markings for accurate measurements.

3. Meal Prep Containers: Having a set of meal prep containers allows you to portion and store your meals conveniently. Look for containers that are microwave-safe, dishwasher-safe, and leak-proof.

4. Blender or Food Processor: A blender or food processor is useful for creating smoothies, protein shakes, and homemade sauces. It can help you incorporate ingredients with specific macros and achieve desired textures.

5. Spiralizer: A spiralizer is a handy tool for creating vegetable noodles or "zoodles" from zucchini, carrots, or sweet potatoes. It's a great way to substitute traditional pasta with low-carb, high-fiber options.

6. Steamer Basket: A steamer basket is ideal for cooking vegetables while preserving their nutrients. Steamed vegetables can be a nutritious addition to your macro meals.

7. Grill Pan or Grill: Grilling is a healthy cooking method that adds flavor to your proteins and vegetables without adding excess fat. Invest in a grill pan or an outdoor grill to prepare grilled chicken, steak, fish, and grilled vegetables.

8. Non-Stick Cooking Spray: Non-stick cooking spray helps reduce the need for added fats when cooking. It allows you to minimize calories while preventing ingredients from sticking to the pan.

9. Air Fryer: An air fryer is a versatile appliance that can crisp up foods with minimal oil. It's perfect for preparing crispy chicken tenders, roasted vegetables, or sweet potato fries while reducing added fats.

10. Herb and Spice Grinder: Fresh herbs and spices can add flavor to your macro meals without adding significant calories. Invest in a herb and spice grinder to freshly grind your favorite seasonings.

11. Oven-Safe Meat Thermometer: An oven-safe meat thermometer ensures that your proteins are cooked to the desired temperature without overcooking. This helps maintain the juiciness and texture of your meats.

12. Immersion Blender: An immersion blender is a handheld tool that allows you to blend soups and sauces directly in the pot. It's convenient for creating smooth textures without transferring ingredients to a separate blender.

13. Kitchen Timer: A kitchen timer ensures accurate cooking times and prevents overcooking or undercooking your meals. You can use a traditional timer or opt for a digital version on your phone or smart device.

14. Salad Spinner: A salad spinner enables you to wash and dry your leafy greens thoroughly. It's a useful tool for preparing fresh salads that are rich in fiber and low in calories.

15. Food Storage Bags: Zip-top food storage bags are helpful for portioning and freezing ingredients **in** individual servings. They allow you to prepare meals in advance and easily track your macros.

16. Mandoline Slicer: A mandoline slicer helps you achieve consistent and thin slices of fruits and vegetables. It's useful for creating uniform slices for salads, gratins, or vegetable chips.

17. Nut Milk Bag: If you enjoy making your own nut milk or straining homemade sauces, a nut milk bag is essential. It helps separate the liquid from the solids, resulting in smooth and creamy textures.

18. Portion Control Plates: Portion control plates have designated sections for different food groups, promoting balanced meals and portion awareness. Using these plates can assist you in managing your macros effectively.

19. Water Bottle with Measurements: Staying hydrated is crucial on a macro diet. Having a water bottle with measurements can help you track your water intake and stay on top of your hydration goals.

20. Macro Tracking App: While not a physical tool, a macro tracking app is invaluable for monitoring your macronutrient intake. It allows you to log your meals, scan barcodes, and track your progress toward your macro goals.

Remember, these tools are meant to enhance your macro meal preparation experience, but they are not mandatory. Choose tools based on your preferences.

The following is-friendly ingredients;

1. Whole Grains:

Incorporating whole grains into your pantry is essential for a balanced diet. Opt for options like brown rice, quinoa, oats, whole wheat pasta, and whole grain bread. It produces complex carbohydrates, fiber, and essential nutrients.

2. Lean Proteins:

Including lean protein sources in your pantry is crucial for muscle repair and growth. Stock up on items such as canned tuna, salmon, chicken breast, turkey breast, beans, lentils, and tofu. These options offer a good balance of protein while being lower in fat.

3. Healthy Fats:

Including healthy fats in your pantry is important for overall health and satiety. Choose items like extra virgin olive oil, avocado oil, coconut oil, nuts (almonds, walnuts, cashews), seeds (chia seeds, flaxseeds), and nut butter (peanut butter, almond butter). They are rich in omega-3 fatty acids and provide essential nutrients.

4. Fresh and Frozen Produce:

Stocking your pantry with fresh and frozen fruits and vegetables ensures that you always have nutrient-dense options available. Choose a variety of colorful options like spinach, kale, broccoli, berries, apples, oranges, and frozen mixed vegetables. It provides fiber, vitamins, minerals, and antioxidants.

5. Low-Sugar Condiments and Sauces:

Many condiments and sauces can be high in added sugars, so it's important to choose options that are macro-friendly. Look for low-sugar or sugar-free options like mustard, hot sauce, salsa, low-sodium soy sauce, balsamic vinegar, and spices. These add flavor to your meals without adding unnecessary calories.

6. Herbs and Spices:

Building a collection of herbs and spices in your pantry is an excellent way to enhance the flavors of your dishes without relying on added fats or sugars. Stock up on essentials like garlic powder, onion powder, cumin, paprika, turmeric, cinnamon, and dried herbs.

7. Healthy Sweeteners:

If you have a sweet tooth, it's good to have some macro-friendly sweeteners on hand. Opt for options like stevia, monk fruit, or erythritol, which are low in calories and have minimal impact on blood sugar levels. These can be used in baking or to sweeten beverages without adding excessive calories.

8. Canned Goods:

Canned goods are convenient and can be stored for a long time. Choose options like canned tomatoes, beans, lentils, and coconut milk (light version). These can be used in various recipes, such as soups, stews, and sauces, to add flavor, fiber, and protein.

9. Healthy Snacks:

It's important to have macro-friendly snacks readily available to avoid reaching for unhealthy options. Stock up on items like protein bars, Greek yogurt, rice cakes, air-popped popcorn, and jerky (lean meat or vegetarian options). These provide a quick and convenient source of protein and energy.

10. Hydration:

While not technically a pantry item, staying hydrated is vital for overall health. Keep a supply of water bottles or a water filtration system to ensure you have easy access to clean, refreshing water throughout the day.

Therefore, remember to regularly check expiration dates and rotate your pantry items to maintain freshness. By stocking your pantry with macro-friendly ingredients, you'll be well-equipped to prepare nutritious and balanced meals that support your health and fitness goals.

Making smart grocery shopping choices for a macro diet involves selecting foods that align with your macronutrient goals while providing essential nutrients. Here are some tips to help you make wise choices at the grocery store:

1. Plan Ahead:

Before heading to the grocery store, plan your meals for the week. It helps you to determine what ingredients you need and prevent impulse purchases.

2. Stick to the Perimeter:

The perimeter of the grocery store is typically where you'll find fresh produce, lean proteins, and dairy products. Focus on filling your cart with these whole foods, as they are often the foundation of a macro diet.

3. Read Food Labels:

Pay close attention to the nutritional information on food labels. Look for products that are low in added sugars, saturated fats, and sodium. Aim for foods that are high in protein and fiber, as these nutrients are essential for a macro diet.

4. Choose Lean Proteins:

Opt for lean protein sources like skinless chicken breast, turkey, lean cuts of beef, fish, tofu, tempeh, and legumes. It provides high-quality protein while being relatively low in fat.

5. Select Whole Grains:

Include whole grains in your cart, such as brown rice, quinoa, oats, whole wheat bread, and whole wheat pasta. These complex carbohydrates provide fiber and are more nutrient-dense compared to refined grains.

6. Load Up on Fruits and Vegetables:

Fill your cart with a variety of fresh or frozen fruits and vegetables. These nutrient-rich foods are low in calories and high in fiber, vitamins, minerals, and antioxidants.

7. Choose Healthy Fats:

Opt for sources of healthy fats, such as avocados, nuts, seeds, olive oil, and fatty fish like salmon. These fats produce essential fatty acids and contribute to satiety.

8. Be Mindful of Condiments:

Many condiments can be high in added sugars, unhealthy fats, and sodium. Read labels and opt for healthier alternatives like mustard, hot sauce, low-sugar ketchup, and homemade dressings using olive oil and vinegar.

9. Stock Up on Greek Yogurt and Cottage Cheese:

Greek yogurt and cottage cheese are excellent sources of protein and can be versatile in meal preparation. Look for options that are low in added sugars and choose plain varieties that you can flavor yourself.

10. Minimize Processed Foods:

Try to limit processed foods like sugary snacks, packaged meals, and sugary drinks. These tend to be high in added sugars, unhealthy fats, and empty calories.

11. Don't Forget Hydration:

Remember to include water on your grocery list. Hydration is important for overall health and can help with appetite control. Consider adding sparkling water or herbal teas for its variety.

By following these tips, you'll make smarter grocery shopping choices that align with your macro diet and support your health and fitness goals. Remember to stay consistent and make gradual adjustments to your shopping list as you learn more about your specific macronutrient needs.

CHAPTER 4:

MEAL PLANNING MADE EASY

-THE ART OF MEAL PREPPING

Meal prepping is a popular strategy used by many individuals following a macro diet to stay on track with their nutrition goals. It involves planning, preparing, and portioning meals in advance, typically for a week, to ensure that you have healthy and balanced meals readily available throughout the week. This approach not only saves time and reduces stress but also helps you maintain control over your macronutrient intake.

Macro diet, short for macronutrient diet, focuses on the balance of macronutrients—carbohydrates, proteins, and fats—in your meals. It emphasizes consuming specific ratios of these macronutrients to support various health and fitness goals, such as weight loss, muscle gain, or overall well-being. Meal prepping for a macro diet involves careful consideration of these macronutrient ratios to ensure that each meal meets your dietary requirements.

Here are some key steps to effectively meal prep for a macro diet:

1. Set Your Macronutrient Goals: Determine your specific macronutrient ratios based on your goals and dietary preferences. Common ratios include the balanced 40% carbohydrates, 30% protein, and 30% fat, as well as other variations depending on your needs.

2. Plan Your Meals: Create a meal plan for the week, considering your macronutrient goals. Include a variety of protein sources (such as lean meats, poultry, fish, tofu, or legumes), complex carbohydrates (like whole grains, sweet potatoes, or quinoa), and healthy fats (such as avocado, nuts, seeds, or olive oil). Incorporate a range of vegetables and fruits for added nutrients and fiber.

3. Grocery Shopping: Make a detailed grocery list based on your meal plan. Ensure you have all the necessary ingredients to prepare your meals. Opt for fresh and whole foods whenever possible to maximize nutritional value.

4. Prep and Cook: Dedicate a specific time for meal prepping, such as a weekend day or a day off. Start by washing and chopping vegetables, cooking grains, and proteins. Then portion out your meals into individual containers, keeping the macronutrient ratios in mind. Label each container with the meal and day of the week to stay organized.

5. Storage and Freezing: Proper storage is crucial to maintain food quality and safety. Refrigerate meals that will be consumed within the first few days. For meals that will be eaten later in the week, consider freezing them to preserve freshness. Use freezer bags to prevent freezer burn and maintain flavor.

6. Variety and Flexibility: While meal prepping, aim for variety to prevent boredom and ensure you receive a wide range of nutrients. Consider rotating different proteins, vegetables, and grains throughout the week. Additionally, allow for some flexibility in your meal plan to accommodate unexpected changes or cravings.

7. Portion Control: Pay attention to portion sizes to ensure you're consuming the right amount of each macronutrient. Use measuring cups, a food scale, or pre-portioned containers to maintain accuracy. This step is crucial for achieving your desired macronutrient ratios and managing calorie intake.

8. Reheating and Enjoying: When it's time to eat your prepped meals, reheat them thoroughly to ensure food safety. Follow the appropriate reheating instructions for each dish to maintain taste and texture. Enjoy your meals mindfully, savoring the flavors and appreciating the effort you put into your macro diet.

Meal prepping for a macro diet provides several benefits, which include;

1. Time Savings: By prepping meals in advance, you save time throughout the week, as you won't need to cook every day or make last-minute food decisions.

2. Portion Control: Meal prepping helps you maintain portion control, which is essential for managing your macronutrient intake and reaching your goals.

3. Consistency: Following a macro diet requires consistency. Meal prepping ensures that you have nutritious meals readily available, reducing the temptation to make less healthy choices.

4. Cost-Effective: By planning your meals and buying ingredients in bulk, you can save money in the long run. It also reduces the likelihood of food waste since you only buy what you need.

5. Reduced Stress: Having your meals prepared in advance eliminates the stress of deciding what to eat and cooking from scratch when you're busy or tired.

However, meal prepping is a flexible process that can be tailored to your personal preferences and schedule. Use different recipes, flavors, and cooking methods to keep your meals exciting and enjoyable. With consistency and a well-planned macro diet, meal prepping can be a powerful tool to support your health and fitness goals.

-BALANCING MACROS ACROSS YOUR MEALS

Balancing macros across your meals is a crucial aspect of maintaining a healthy and well-rounded diet. Macros, short for macronutrients, refer to carbohydrates, proteins, and fats—the three primary nutrients that provide energy to the body. Achieving an appropriate balance of these macronutrients in your meals helps support optimal nutrition, energy levels, and overall well-being. Here are some effective ways to balance macros across your meals:

1. Determine your macronutrient needs: Before you can balance your macros, it's important to understand your individual macronutrient requirements. Factors such as age, gender, activity level, and specific goals (such as weight loss, muscle building, or general maintenance) can influence your ideal macronutrient ratios. Consulting with a registered dietitian or using online calculators can help you establish your personalized macronutrient goals.

2. Prioritize lean proteins: Incorporating a sufficient amount of protein into your meals is essential for various bodily functions, including muscle repair and growth, hormone production, and satiety. Opt for lean protein sources such as chicken, turkey, fish, tofu, beans, lentils, and Greek yogurt. Aim to include a serving of protein with each meal.

3. Include complex carbohydrates: Complex carbohydrates provide sustained energy and fiber, which aids in digestion and helps you feel full. Prioritize whole grains like brown rice, quinoa, whole wheat bread, and oats. Additionally, include a variety of fruits, vegetables, and legumes, as they offer valuable nutrients and fiber.

4. Incorporate healthy fats: While fats should be consumed in moderation, they play a vital role in hormone regulation, nutrient absorption, and brain function. Opt for healthy fats like avocados, nuts, seeds, olive oil, and fatty fish (such as salmon or mackerel). Be mindful of portion sizes since fats are calorie-dense.

5. Pay attention to portion control: Even when selecting nutritious foods, portion control is essential. Maintain a balanced approach by including appropriate portions of each macronutrient group. A simple guideline is to fill half of your plate with vegetables, allocate a quarter to lean protein, and reserve the remaining quarter for complex carbohydrates or healthy fats.

6. Plan your meals in advance: By planning your meals ahead of time, you can ensure a balanced macro distribution throughout the day. Consider using meal planning apps or spreadsheets to organize your meals and track your macros. This approach can help you make intentional choices and avoid haphazardly consuming imbalanced meals.

7. Monitor your intake: Keeping track of your macronutrient intake can be helpful, especially when you're starting to balance your macros. There are various mobile apps and online tools available that can assist you in monitoring and adjusting your macronutrient ratios based on your goals.

8. Listen to your body: While macronutrient balance is important, it's crucial to listen to your body's unique needs and preferences. Pay attention to how different macronutrient ratios make you feel and perform. Try out various minor modifications to see what suits you the best.

Achieving a balanced macro distribution doesn't mean obsessing over every meal. Instead, aim for consistency and long-term sustainability. Balancing macros across your meals is a flexible approach that can be tailored to your individual needs and preferences, promoting a healthier and more enjoyable eating experience.

-CREATING WEEKLY MEAL PLANS

Creating weekly meal plans for a macro diet involves strategically balancing your macronutrient intake to meet your specific goals. By focusing on the right proportions of carbohydrates, proteins, and fats, you can optimize your nutrition and support your fitness objectives. Here's a step-by-step guide to help you create your weekly meal plans for a macro diet:

1. Determine Your Goals: Before you start planning your meals, it's essential to define your goals. Whether you want to lose weight, gain muscle, or maintain your current physique, understanding your objectives will guide your macro distribution.

2. Calculate Your Calorie Intake: To create a baseline for your meal plans, determine your daily calorie needs. Several online calculators can assist you in estimating your total daily energy expenditure (TDEE) based on factors such as age, gender, weight, height, and activity level. This TDEE will serve as a starting point for adjusting your macro proportions.

3. Set Your Macro Ratios: Once you have your calorie intake, you need to establish your macro ratios. The most common macronutrient breakdowns are:
- Carbohydrates: 45-65% of total calories
- Proteins: 10-35% of total calories
- Fats: 20-35% of total calories
These ranges can be adjusted based on your specific goals and preferences. For example, a higher protein intake might be suitable for muscle building, while a lower carbohydrate intake could be helpful for weight loss.

4. Calculate Your Macro Targets: Using your calorie intake and desired macro ratios, calculate your specific macro targets. Start by multiplying the total calories by the percentage allocated to each macronutrient. Then, divide the resulting value by the calorie content per gram of each macronutrient:
- Carbohydrates: 4 calories per gram
- Proteins: 4 calories per gram
- Fats: 9 calories per gram
This calculation will give you the number of grams of each macronutrient you should aim for daily.

5. Choose a Meal Planning Method: There are various approaches to meal planning. Some people prefer prepping meals in advance for the entire week, while others opt for daily meal planning. Select a method that suits your schedule, lifestyle, and personal preferences.

6. Plan Balanced Meals: When creating your weekly meal plans, aim for balanced meals that include a variety of nutrient-dense foods. Incorporate lean proteins, whole grains, fruits, vegetables, healthy fats, and legumes in your diet. Choose foods that you enjoy and that align with your macro targets.

7. Track Your Food Intake: To ensure you're meeting your macro targets, track your food intake using a reliable tracking app or journal. Hence, it will help you stay accountable and make adjustments if necessary. Many mobile apps make tracking macros and calories easy by providing extensive food databases.

8. Plan for Flexibility: While it's important to stick to your macro goals, it's also crucial to allow for flexibility in your meal plans. Incorporate some variety and include foods you love to avoid feeling deprived. Always remember that sustainability is key to long-term success.

9. Seek Professional Guidance: If you're new to macro dieting or have specific health concerns, it's advisable to consult with a registered dietitian or nutritionist. They can provide personalized guidance, help you set appropriate macro targets, and ensure you're meeting your nutritional needs.

10. Monitor and Adjust: Regularly assess your progress and make adjustments as needed. Your macro targets may need to be tweaked based on your body's response and changes in your goals or activity levels.

- TIPS FOR ORGANIZING AND STORING MEALS

Organizing and storing meals is essential when following a macro diet, as it helps you stay on track with your nutrition goals and makes mealtime more convenient. Here are some tips to help you effectively organize and store your meals while following a macro diet:

1. Meal Planning: Start by creating a meal plan for the week. This involves deciding on the meals you'll have each day and calculating their macronutrient content. Look for recipes that fit your macro ratios and ensure they include a good balance of proteins, carbohydrates, and healthy fats.

2. Batch Cooking: Consider batch cooking your meals in advance. This involves preparing larger quantities of food and dividing them into individual portions. By doing this, you save time and effort throughout the week, as you'll have pre-portioned meals ready to go.

3. Portion Control: Use food scales or measuring cups to accurately portion your meals according to your macro goals. This helps you maintain consistency and ensures you're consuming the desired amount of each macronutrient.

4. Meal Prep Containers: Invest in high-quality, BPA-free meal prep containers. Look for containers with separate compartments to keep different food items separate, preventing them from getting soggy or mixing together. It equally makes it easier to store and transport your meals.

5. Labeling: Clearly label your meal prep containers with the date and contents. This helps you keep track of the freshness of your meals and prevents any confusion when selecting a meal to eat.

6. Freezing Meals: If you're batch cooking or preparing meals ahead of time, consider freezing some of them. Freezing meals extends their shelf life, allowing you to enjoy them later without worrying about spoilage. Ensure to use freezer-safe containers to prevent freezer burn.

7. Refrigeration: For meals that you'll consume within a few days, store them in the refrigerator. Keep perishable foods at or below 40°F (4°C) to maintain their freshness and minimize the risk of bacterial growth. Make sure to consume refrigerated meals within the recommended storage time frames to avoid spoilage.

8. Organize Your Fridge: Keep your fridge well-organized to easily locate and access your prepped meals. Designate a specific area or shelf for

your meal prep containers, making it easier to grab
and go when needed.

9. Portable Snacks: Prepare portable macro-friendly snacks that you can easily grab when you're on the go. Examples include protein bars, hard-boiled eggs, Greek yogurt cups, pre-cut vegetables, and nuts. Having these options readily available helps you stick to your diet even when you're away from home.

10. Tracking Apps: Utilize nutrition tracking apps or online tools to monitor your macro intake accurately. These apps can help you calculate and log the macronutrient content of your meals, making it easier to stay within your target ranges.

By following these tips for organizing and storing meals in a macro diet, you can save time, stay on track with your nutrition goals, and ensure that you have healthy, balanced meals readily available whenever you need them. Remember, consistency is key, and effective meal organization and storage can greatly contribute to your success on a macro diet.

CHAPTER 5:

BREAKFAST DELIGHTS

-ENERGIZING AND PROTEIN-PACKED BREAKFAST RECIPES

When following a macro diet, it's important to start your day with a breakfast that provides energy and is packed with protein to support your fitness and nutrition goals. Here are some energizing and protein-packed breakfast recipes that are perfect for a macro diet:

1. Protein Pancakes:
Ingredients:
- 1 scoop of protein powder (flavor of your choice)
- 1/2 cup of oats
- 1/2 cup of cottage cheese
- 2 egg whites
- 1/2 teaspoon of baking powder
- Optional toppings: fresh berries, sliced banana, nut butter

Instructions:
- In a blender, combine protein powder, oats, cottage cheese, egg whites, and baking powder. Blend until smooth.
- Heat a non-stick pan over medium heat and spray with cooking spray.

- put the pancake batter onto the pan to form small pancakes.
- Cook each side till it turns golden brown.
- Serve with your favorite toppings.

2. Egg and Vegetable Scramble:
Ingredients:
- 2 whole eggs
- 4 egg whites
- 1/2 cup of chopped mixed vegetables (bell peppers, spinach, mushrooms, etc.)
- 1 tablespoon of olive oil
- Salt and pepper to taste

Instructions:
- In a non-stick pan, Heat olive oil over medium heat.
- Add the chopped vegetables and sauté until they are slightly tender.
- In a bowl, whisk together the whole eggs.
- Pour the egg mixture over the sautéed vegetables and cook, stirring occasionally, until the eggs are fully cooked.
- Then add salt and pepper to taste.
- Serve with a side of whole grain toast or avocado slices.

3. Greek Yogurt Parfait:
Ingredients:
- A cup of Greek yogurt (plain or flavored)
- 1/4 cup of granola
- 1/4 cup of mixed berries (strawberries, blueberries, raspberries)
- 1 tablespoon of honey

Instructions:
- In a glass or bowl, layer Greek yogurt, granola, and mixed berries.
- Drizzle honey over the top.
- Use all the ingredients by repeating the layers
- Enjoy as is or refrigerate overnight for a delicious, ready-to-eat breakfast.

4. Protein Smoothie Bowl:
Ingredients:
- 1 scoop of protein powder (flavor of your choice)
- 1 frozen banana
- 1/2 cup of frozen berries (blueberries, raspberries, strawberries)
- 1/2 cup of milk
- Toppings: sliced almonds, chia seeds, shredded coconut, fresh fruit

Instructions:
- In a blender, combine protein powder, frozen banana, frozen berries, and almond milk.
- Blend until smooth and creamy.
- Pour the smoothie into a bowl.
- Add your favorite toppings to enhance texture and flavor.
- Enjoy with a spoon.

5. Quinoa and Egg Bowl:
Ingredients:
- 1/2 cup of cooked quinoa
- 2 boiled eggs, sliced
- 1/4 cup of diced avocado

- 1/4 cup of cherry tomatoes, halved
- 1 tablespoon of chopped fresh herbs (parsley, cilantro, basil)
- Salt and pepper to taste

Instructions:
- In a bowl, combine cooked quinoa, sliced boiled eggs, diced avocado, cherry tomatoes, and fresh herbs.
- Season with salt and pepper.
- Mix well to combine all the ingredients.
- Serve as a nutritious and protein-packed breakfast option.

These breakfast recipes provide a good balance of protein, carbohydrates, and healthy fats, making them suitable for a macro diet. Remember to adjust the quantities of ingredients to fit your specific macro goals. With these energizing and protein-packed breakfast options, you'll kickstart your day with a satisfying meal that fuels your body and supports your fitness journey.

-QUICK AND EASY MAKE-AHEAD OPTIONS; SMOOTHIES, OVERNIGHT OATS, AND EGG DISHES.

When following a macro diet, it can be beneficial to have quick and easy make-ahead options for busy mornings or times when you need a convenient meal. Smoothies, overnight oats, and egg dishes are great choices that can be prepped in advance and customized to fit your macros. Here's an extensive look at these make-ahead options in a macro diet:

1. Smoothies:
Smoothies are an excellent way to pack in nutrients and macros in a quick and convenient manner. Here's how to make them make-ahead friendly:

a. Pre-portioned Smoothie Packs:
- Prepare individual smoothie packs by combining your desired fruits, vegetables, and any other additions like protein powder or nut butter in ziplock bags.
- Store these packs in the freezer.
- When you're ready to make a smoothie, simply grab a pack, add a liquid of your choice (water, milk, or plant-based milk), and blend until smooth.

b. Batch-prepared Smoothies:
- Blend a large batch of smoothie base using your favorite ingredients and adjust the quantities to fit your macros.
- Pour the smoothie into individual containers or ice cube trays if you prefer smaller portions.
- Freeze the containers or trays.
- When you want a smoothie, thaw the container in the fridge overnight or blend the frozen cubes with a liquid of your choice.

2. Overnight Oats:
Overnight oats are great for a quick and filling breakfast that can be made ahead of time. Here's how to prepare them:

a. Basic Overnight Oats:
- In a jar or container, combine rolled oats, your choice of milk or yogurt, and a sweetener like honey or maple syrup.
- Add in toppings like chia seeds, flaxseeds, or protein powder to increase the nutritional value.
- Stir well, cover, and refrigerate overnight.
- In the morning, give it a good stir and enjoy the cold or heat it up if desired.

b. Customizable Overnight Oats:
- Follow the basic overnight oats recipe but experiment with different flavor combinations by adding fruits, nuts, and spices.
- For example, you can add mashed banana, cinnamon, and chopped walnuts for a banana bread flavor, or mix in diced apples and a sprinkle of cinnamon for an apple pie-inspired oat.

3. Egg Dishes:
Eggs are a versatile and protein-rich option for a macro-friendly breakfast. Here are a couple of make-ahead egg dishes:

a. Egg Muffins:
- In a bowl, whisk together eggs, your choice of vegetables (spinach, bell peppers, mushrooms, etc.), cooked lean meats (turkey bacon, chicken sausage), and shredded cheese.
- Add the mixture into greased muffin tins.
- Bake in the oven at 350°F (175°C) for about 15-20 minutes or until the eggs are set.

- Once cooled, store the egg muffins in an airtight
container in the fridge.
- microwave or enjoy it cold.

b. Frittata:
- In a large oven-safe skillet, sauté your choice of
vegetables and protein.
- In a mixing bowl, whisk eggs, milk, and seasonings
together.
- Pour the egg mixture over the sautéed vegetables
and protein in the skillet.
- Let the edges be set, by Cook for a few minutes.
- Transfer the skillet to the oven and bake at 350°F
(175°C) for about 15-20 minutes or until the frittata is
cooked through.
- Allow it to cool, then slice into individual portions and
store in the fridge.

By prepping smoothies, overnight oats, and egg
dishes ahead of time, you can have a variety of quick
and macro-friendly breakfast options at your
fingertips. These make-ahead meals save you time in
the morning while ensuring you start your day with a
nutritious and balanced meal. Feel free to customize
these recipes with your preferred ingredients, making
sure to adjust the quantities to fit your specific macro
goals.

Here's an extensive list of nourishing lunch recipes suitable for a macro diet on busy days:

1. Quinoa Power Bowl:
- Cooked quinoa (complex carbs and protein)
- Grilled chicken or tofu (protein)
- Steamed broccoli and kale (fiber and vitamins)
- Sliced avocado (healthy fats)
- Cherry tomatoes (fiber and antioxidants)
- Dressing: Lemon juice, olive oil, and herbs

2. Mexican-inspired Burrito Bowl:
- Lean ground turkey or black beans (protein)
- Brown rice (complex carbs)
- Mixed bell peppers and onions (fiber and vitamins)
- Corn kernels (fiber and antioxidants)
- Sliced avocado (healthy fats)
- Salsa or homemade pico de gallo

3. Asian-inspired Stir-Fry:
- Thinly sliced chicken, beef, or shrimp (protein)
- Assorted vegetables like broccoli, bell peppers, carrots, and snap peas (fiber and vitamins)
- Brown rice or whole wheat noodles (complex carbs)
- Stir-fry sauce: Low-sodium soy sauce, ginger, garlic, and sesame oil

4. Mediterranean Salad:
- Mixed greens (fiber and vitamins)
- Grilled chicken or chickpeas (protein)

- Cucumber, cherry tomatoes, and bell peppers
(fiber and antioxidants)
- Feta cheese (protein and calcium)
- Kalamata olives (healthy fats)
- Dressing: Olive oil, lemon juice, and herbs like
oregano and basil

5. Tuna and Quinoa Stuffed Bell Peppers:
- Canned tuna (protein)
- Cooked quinoa (complex carbs and protein)
- Diced vegetables like onions, carrots, and zucchini
(fiber and vitamins)
- Tomato sauce or marinara
- Bell peppers as the edible bowl (fiber and
vitamins)

6. Chickpea Salad:
- Canned chickpeas (protein and fiber)
- Diced cucumber, cherry tomatoes, and red onions
(fiber and antioxidants)
- Chopped parsley and mint (fiber and vitamins)
- Lemon juice and olive oil for dressing.

7. Salmon and Sweet Potato:
- Grilled or baked salmon fillet (protein and healthy
fats)
- Baked sweet potato wedges (complex carbs and
fiber)
- Steamed asparagus or broccoli (fiber and
vitamins)
- Lemon-dill sauce: Greek yogurt, lemon juice, dill,
and garlic

8. Lentil Soup:
- Lentils (protein and fiber)
- Carrots, celery, and onions (fiber and vitamins)
- Vegetable broth (low-sodium)
- Herbs and spices such as cumin, turmeric, and paprika

9. Greek Chicken Wrap:
- Grilled chicken breast (protein)
- Whole wheat wrap or pita (complex carbs)
- Tzatziki sauce (Greek yogurt, cucumber, dill, and garlic)
- Sliced tomatoes, cucumbers, and red onions (fiber and vitamins)
- Kalamata olives (healthy fats)

10. Egg and Vegetable Frittata:
- Egg whites or whole eggs (protein)
- Chopped vegetables like spinach, bell peppers, onions, and mushrooms (fiber and vitamins)
- Feta cheese (protein and calcium)
- Baked in muffin tins for easy portion control

Remember to adjust the portion sizes of each ingredient to meet your specific macro goals. These recipes provide a good balance of proteins, complex carbohydrates, healthy fats, and fiber for a nourishing lunch while following a macro diet. Prepare it based on your personal preferences and dietary needs.

Some other Portable and office-friendly meals such as salads, wraps, and grain bowls are great options for those following a macro diet. These meals can be easily prepared in advance and taken with you on-the-go. Some ideas for each categories are as follows;

SALADS:

1. Greek Salad: Combine chopped cucumbers, tomatoes, red onions, olives, and feta cheese. Serve it with olive oil, lemon juice, and oregano.

2. Chicken Caesar Salad: Toss grilled chicken, romaine lettuce, cherry tomatoes, grated Parmesan cheese, and Caesar dressing together.

3. Cobb Salad: Arrange mixed greens, grilled chicken, hard-boiled eggs, avocado, bacon, cherry tomatoes, and blue cheese in a container. Use a vinaigrette dressing on the side.

WRAPS:

1. Veggie Wrap: Spread hummus on a whole-grain tortilla and fill it with sliced cucumbers, bell peppers, carrots, lettuce, and feta cheese. Secure with a toothpick and roll it up.

2. Turkey Club Wrap: Layer sliced turkey, bacon, lettuce, tomato, and mayo on a tortilla. Cut it into bite-sized pieces and Roll it up.

3. Buffalo Chicken Wrap: Mix grilled chicken with buffalo sauce, and add shredded lettuce, diced celery, and ranch dressing. To enjoy, wrap it in a tortilla .

GRAIN BOWLS:

1. Quinoa Bowl: Cook quinoa and top it with grilled chicken or tofu, roasted vegetables, avocado slices, and a drizzle of balsamic vinaigrette.

2. Mexican Rice Bowl: Combine cooked brown rice, black beans, grilled peppers and onions, salsa, guacamole, and shredded cheese. Add a squeeze of lime juice for extra flavor.

3. Teriyaki Salmon Bowl: Cook salmon and serve it on a bed of brown rice with steamed broccoli, sliced carrots, and a drizzle of teriyaki sauce.

Pack these meals in leak-proof containers and keep them refrigerated until you're ready to eat. Enjoy your office-friendly meals.

CHAPTER 7:

SATISFYING DINNERS

-FLAVORFUL AND FILLING DINNER RECIPES.

Here are some flavorful and filling dinner recipes for a macro diet, along with their methods of preparation:

1. Baked Lemon Herb Chicken with Roasted Vegetables:
- Preheat the oven to 400°F (200°C).
- In a small bowl, combine lemon juice, olive oil, minced garlic, dried herbs (such as thyme, rosemary, and oregano), salt, and pepper.
- Place chicken breasts on a baking sheet and brush the lemon herb mixture over them.
- Toss a variety of vegetables (such as carrots, Brussels sprouts, and red onions) in olive oil, salt, and pepper, then spread them around the chicken.
- Bake for about 25-30 minutes or until the chicken is cooked through and the vegetables are tender.

2. Quinoa Stuffed Bell Peppers:
- Adjust the oven's temperature to 190°C, or 375°F.
- Remove the seeds and membranes from bell peppers by cutting off the tops.
- In a skillet, heat olive oil and sauté diced onions, minced garlic, and chopped vegetables (such as zucchini, mushrooms, and spinach).

- In a separate pot, cook quinoa according to package instructions.
- Combine the cooked quinoa with the sautéed vegetables and add salt, pepper, and herbs (such as basil or parsley) to taste.
- Stuff the mixture into the hollowed bell peppers, place them on a baking dish, and bake for 25-30 minutes or until the peppers are tender.

3. Shrimp Stir-Fry with Brown Rice:
- Cook brown rice according to package instructions.
- In a wok or large skillet, heat sesame oil and sauté minced garlic, grated ginger, and thinly sliced vegetables (such as bell peppers, snap peas, and carrots).
- Place the peeled and deveined shrimp in the skillet and heat them until they become pink and are thoroughly done.
- Season with soy sauce or tamari, a touch of honey or maple syrup, and a sprinkle of red pepper flakes (optional).
- Serve the stir-fry over the cooked brown rice.

4. Veggie-Packed Turkey Chili:
- In a large pot or Dutch oven, heat olive oil and sauté diced onions, minced garlic, and chopped bell peppers until softened.
- Add ground turkey and cook until browned.
- Stir in tomato paste, diced tomatoes, drained and rinsed beans (such as black beans and kidney beans), and spices (such as chili powder, cumin, paprika, and oregano).

- Allow the flavors to combine by simmering the chili
for 20 to 30 minutes.
- Serve the chili hot, and top with diced avocado,
chopped cilantro, and a dollop of Greek yogurt.

5. Salmon and Asparagus Foil Packets:
- Preheat the oven to 400°F (200°C).
- Place a salmon filet on a large piece of aluminum
foil.
- Season the salmon with salt, pepper, minced
garlic, and a squeeze of lemon juice.
- Arrange trimmed asparagus spears around the
salmon.
- Fold the edges of the foil to create a sealed
packet, ensuring it is tightly closed.
- Bake the foil packets for approximately 15-20
minutes or until the salmon is cooked to your desired
doneness.

However, Feel free to modify the recipes by adding or
substituting ingredients based on your preferences,
dietary restrictions, or seasonal availability. Enjoy your
flavorful and filling macro-friendly dinners

**-OTHERS INCLUDE ONE-POT MEALS AND SHEET
PAN DINNERS FOR VEGETARIAN, POULTRY,
SEAFOOD, AND LEAN MEAT OPTIONS.**

One-pot meals and sheet pan dinners are not only
convenient but also great options for those following a
macro diet. They allow you to combine multiple
ingredients in a single cooking vessel, minimizing
cleanup while maximizing flavor and nutrition. Here

are some ideas for one-pot meals and sheet pan dinners with vegetarian, poultry, seafood, and lean meat options that align with a macro diet:

1. One-Pot Quinoa and Vegetable Stir-Fry (Vegetarian):

- In a large skillet or wok, heat olive oil and sauté diced onions and minced garlic until softened.
- Add chopped vegetables like bell peppers, broccoli, snap peas, and carrots, and cook until slightly tender.
- Stir in cooked quinoa and season with soy sauce or tamari, ginger, and a touch of honey or maple syrup.
- Optionally, you can add scrambled eggs or tofu for extra protein.
- Stir and cook for a few more minutes, or until everything is fully heated.
- Garnish with chopped green onions and toasted sesame seeds, if desired.

2. Sheet Pan Lemon Herb Chicken with Roasted Vegetables (Poultry):

- Preheat the oven to 425°F (220°C).
- On a large sheet pan, arrange chicken breast or thighs and surround them with a mix of chopped vegetables such as sweet potatoes, Brussels sprouts, and red onions.
- Drizzle olive oil over the chicken and vegetables, then season with lemon zest, dried herbs (such as thyme, rosemary, and oregano), salt, and pepper.
- Toss everything together to coat evenly, then spread out in a single layer.

- Roast for about 25-30 minutes or until the chicken is cooked through and the vegetables are golden and tender.

3. One-Pot Shrimp and Vegetable Curry (Seafood):

- In a large pot or deep skillet, heat coconut oil and sauté diced onions until translucent.
- Add minced garlic, grated ginger, and curry paste or powder, and cook for a minute until fragrant.
- Stir in chopped vegetables like bell peppers, zucchini, and cauliflower, and cook for a few minutes.
- When the vegetable broth and coconut milk are added, boil the mixture.
- Add peeled and deveined shrimp and cook until they turn pink and are cooked through.
- Add some salt, pepper, and lime juice for seasoning.
- Serve the curry over cooked brown rice or cauliflower rice.

4. Sheet Pan Baked Salmon with Roasted Asparagus (Seafood):

- Preheat the oven to 425°F (220°C).
- Place salmon filets on a parchment-lined sheet pan and season with salt, pepper, and minced garlic.
- Arrange trimmed asparagus spears around the salmon.
- Drizzle with olive oil and sprinkle with lemon zest and a squeeze of lemon juice.
- Bake for about 12-15 minutes or until the salmon is cooked to your preferred doneness and the asparagus is tender-crisp.

5. One-Pot Turkey and Vegetable Chili (Lean Meat):

- In a large pot or Dutch oven, heat olive oil and
sauté diced onions until softened.
- Add ground turkey and cook until browned.
- Stir in tomato paste, diced tomatoes, drained and
rinsed beans (such as black beans and kidney
beans), chopped bell peppers, and spices like chili
powder, cumin, paprika, and oregano.
-To allow the flavors to blend, simmer the chili for 20
to 30 minutes.
- Add pepper and salt to taste.
- Serve the chili hot, and optionally top with Greek
yogurt, diced avocado, and chopped cilantro.

These one-pot meals and sheet pan dinners offer a
variety of options for different dietary preferences
while providing a balance of macronutrients.
Remember to adjust the portion sizes and ingredients
to meet your specific macro goals. Experiment with
different vegetables, herbs, and spices to suit your
taste preferences and enjoy the simplicity and
deliciousness of these easy-to-make meals.

CHAPTER 8:

SNACKS AND DESSERTS

-GUT-FREE SNACK OPTIONS.

Snacks and desserts are delightful indulgences that can satisfy our cravings and provide us with a moment of pleasure. However, when following a macro diet, it's essential to choose guilt-free snack options that align with your nutritional goals. Here are some ideas for macro-friendly snacks and desserts:

1. Greek Yogurt Parfait: Greek yogurt is packed with protein and can be combined with fruits, nuts, and a drizzle of honey or a sprinkle of granola for added flavor and texture.

2. Rice Cakes with Nut Butter: Opt for whole grain rice cakes and top them with a tablespoon of almond butter or peanut butter. A balance of protein, healthy fats, and carbohydrates is provided by this combination.

3. Veggie Sticks with Hummus: Carrot sticks, celery, cucumber, and bell pepper slices are low in calories and high in fiber. Pair them with a portion-controlled serving of hummus for a satisfying and nutritious snack.

4. Protein Bars: Look for protein bars that have a good balance of macronutrients, including protein, carbohydrates, and healthy fats. Read the labels to ensure they fit your macro goals.

5. Homemade Trail Mix: Create your own trail mix by combining a variety of nuts, seeds, and dried fruits. Be cautious of portion quantities as nuts are calorie-dense.

6. Baked Sweet Potato Fries: Slice sweet potatoes into thin strips, season them with herbs and spices, and bake them until crispy. Sweet potatoes are a great source of carbohydrates and provide essential nutrients.

7. Dark Chocolate: Choose dark chocolate with a high percentage of cocoa (70% or more) as it contains less sugar. Enjoy a small piece or two to satisfy your sweet tooth.

8. Chia Seed Pudding: Combine chia seeds with your choice of milk (such as almond or coconut milk), a natural sweetener like stevia or honey, and flavorings such as vanilla or cocoa powder. Let it sit overnight in the refrigerator for a creamy and nutritious pudding.

It's essential to be mindful of your serving sizes and adjust these snack options to fit your specific macronutrient needs. Consulting with a registered dietitian can provide personalized guidance and help you optimize your macro-friendly snacking choices.

Furthermore, Here are some guilt-free snack options for a macro diet along with their recipes and preparations:

1. Protein Energy Balls:
Ingredients:
- 1 cup rolled oats
- 1/2 cup protein powder (flavor of your choice)
- 1/4 cup nut butter (such as almond or peanut butter)
- 1/4 cup honey or maple syrup
- 1/4 cup unsweetened shredded coconut
- 1/4 cup mini chocolate chips (optional)

Preparation:
1. In a mixing bowl, combine rolled oats, protein powder, nut butter, honey or maple syrup, shredded coconut, and chocolate chips (if using).
2. Stir well until all the ingredients are evenly mixed.
3. Form the mixture into tiny balls with a diameter of approximately an inch.
4. Transfer the balls to a parchment paper-lined baking sheet.
5. Refrigerate for at least 30 minutes to allow the balls to firm up.
6. Once chilled, the protein energy balls are ready to be enjoyed. They can be kept in the fridge for up to a week if they are kept in an airtight container.

2. Veggie and Hummus Wraps:
Ingredients:
- Whole grain tortillas or wraps

- Assorted vegetables (such as lettuce, spinach,
sliced cucumber, shredded carrots, and bell peppers)
- Hummus (flavor of your choice)

Preparation:
1. Lay the tortilla or wrap flat on a clean surface.
2. Spread a generous amount of hummus over the
tortilla.
3. Layer the assorted vegetables evenly on top of the
hummus.
4. Roll the tortilla tightly, tucking in the sides as you
go.
5. Slice the wrap into smaller portions, if desired.
6. Serve immediately or wrap in foil for later
consumption.

3. Greek Yogurt Bark:
Ingredients:
- 2 cups Greek yogurt
- 1 tablespoon honey or maple syrup
- Assorted toppings (such as sliced fruits, nuts, seeds,
or dark chocolate chips)

Preparation:
1. In a bowl, mix the Greek yogurt and honey or
maple syrup until well combined.
2. Use parchment paper to line a baking sheet.
3. Pour the yogurt mixture onto the prepared baking
sheet and spread it evenly with a spatula.
4. Sprinkle your choice of toppings over the yogurt,
pressing them gently to ensure they stick.
5. Place the baking sheet in the freezer for at least 2
hours or until the yogurt bark is completely frozen.

6. Once frozen, break the bark into smaller pieces and store them in an airtight container in the freezer.

4. Baked Kale Chips:
Ingredients:
- Fresh kale leaves, washed and dried
- Olive oil
- Sea salt or seasoning of your choice (such as paprika or garlic powder)

Preparation:
1. Preheat the oven to 300°F (150°C).
2. Tear the kale leaves into bite-sized pieces, discarding the tough stems.
3. Place the kale pieces in a bowl and drizzle with olive oil. Toss to coat the leaves evenly.
4. Arrange the kale on a baking sheet lined with parchment paper, making sure they are spread out in a single layer.
5. Sprinkle sea salt or your preferred seasoning over the kale.
6. Bake for about 10-15 minutes until the kale becomes crispy and slightly browned.
7. Allow the chips to cool before serving. Store any leftovers in an airtight container.

-SWEET TREATS THAT FIT YOUR MACROS AND HOMEMADE PROTEIN BARS AND ENERGY BITES.

Sweet treats that fit your macros can be a delightful addition to your diet while still aligning with your nutritional goals. Homemade protein bars and energy bites are excellent options as they allow you to control

the ingredients and customize them to your liking.
Here are some recipes and preparations for these
delicious and macro-friendly treats:

1. Homemade Protein Bars:
Ingredients:
- 2 cups rolled oats
- 1 cup protein powder (flavor of your choice)
- 1/2 cup nut butter (such as almond or peanut butter)
- 1/4 cup honey or maple syrup
- 1/4 cup unsweetened almond milk (or any milk of
your choice)
- 1/4 cup chopped nuts or seeds (optional)
- 1/4 cup dried fruits (such as cranberries or raisins)
(optional)

Preparation:
1. In a large mixing bowl, combine rolled oats, protein
powder, nut butter, honey or maple syrup, almond
milk, chopped nuts or seeds, and dried fruits (if
using).
2. Stir well until all the ingredients are thoroughly
mixed and form a sticky dough-like consistency.
3. Transfer the mixture into a lined baking dish and
press it down firmly to create an even layer.
4. Place the dish in the refrigerator for at least 1-2
hours to allow the bars to set.
5. Once firm, remove the mixture from the dish and
cut it into bars of your desired size.
6. Store the protein bars in an airtight container in the
refrigerator for up to a week.

2. Homemade Energy Bites:

Ingredients:
- 1 cup rolled oats
- 1/2 cup nut butter (such as almond or peanut butter)
- 1/4 cup honey or maple syrup
- 1/4 cup ground flaxseed or chia seeds
- 1/4 cup dried fruits or tiny chocolate chips, (if desired)
- 1 teaspoon vanilla extract

Preparation:
1. In a mixing bowl, combine rolled oats, nut butter, honey or maple syrup, ground flaxseed or chia seeds, mini chocolate chips or dried fruits (if using), and vanilla extract.
2. Stir well until all the ingredients are thoroughly mixed and form a sticky dough-like consistency.
3. Using your hands or a cookie scoop, roll the mixture into small bite-sized balls.
4. Place the energy bites on a baking sheet lined with parchment paper.
5. Refrigerate for at least 30 minutes to allow the bites to firm up.
6. Once chilled, the energy bites are ready to be enjoyed. Keep them refrigerated for up to a week in an airtight container.

These homemade protein bars and energy bites provide a balance of macronutrients, including protein, carbohydrates, and healthy fats. They can be customized by adding different flavors, such as cocoa powder, spices, or extracts, to suit your taste preferences.

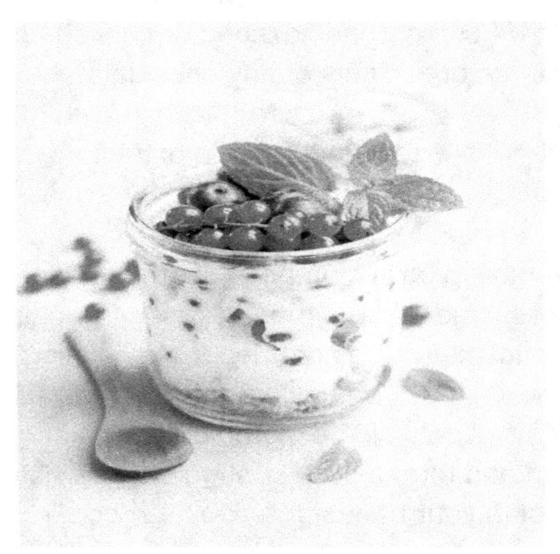

CHAPTER 9:

MACRO MANAGEMENT FOR HEALTH

Managing macros for specific health conditions involves tailoring your nutritional intake to support your health needs. For conditions like diabetes, it's crucial to focus on controlling blood sugar levels. Emphasize complex carbohydrates with a low glycemic index, such as whole grains and legumes, to provide sustained energy.

For cardiovascular health, consider a balanced ratio of fats, prioritizing unsaturated fats from sources like avocados and olive oil. Limit saturated and trans fats, commonly found in processed foods. Adequate intake of omega-3 fatty acids, found in fatty fish and flaxseeds, can also benefit heart health.

In the context of autoimmune disorders, like rheumatoid arthritis, an anti-inflammatory diet may be beneficial. Incorporate foods rich in antioxidants, such as fruits and vegetables, to help manage inflammation. Omega-3 fatty acids and turmeric are also known for their anti-inflammatory properties.

Those with kidney issues should pay attention to protein intake. Adjusting the type and amount of protein may be necessary to reduce the strain on the kidneys. Include high-quality protein sources like lean meats, eggs, and dairy in moderation.Tailoring macros for weight management involves considering the individual's goals. For weight loss, a calorie deficit is essential, but it's equally important to ensure sufficient protein intake to preserve muscle mass. Foods high in fiber might help you feel satisfied.

Individuals with celiac disease or gluten sensitivity need to manage their carbohydrate intake carefully. Opt for gluten-free grains like quinoa and rice, and choose gluten-free alternatives for processed foods.

In the context of managing macros for mental health, consider the impact of nutrition on mood and cognitive function. Omega-3 fatty acids, found in fish and walnuts, may contribute to mental well-being. Additionally, maintaining stable blood sugar levels through balanced macronutrient intake can help regulate mood. It's crucial to note that individual responses to dietary changes vary. Consulting with a healthcare professional or a registered dietitian is advisable to create a personalized plan that aligns with specific health conditions and individual needs.

- ADAPTING THE MACRO DIET FOR VEGETARIAN OR VEGAN LIFESTYLES.

Adapting the macro diet for vegetarian or vegan lifestyles requires careful consideration of nutrient intake to ensure a balanced and healthy diet. The macro diet, also known as flexible dieting, focuses on tracking macronutrients, which include carbohydrates, proteins, and fats, to achieve specific health and fitness goals. While traditionally the macro diet incorporates animal-based protein sources, it is entirely possible to follow this diet as a vegetarian or vegan by making appropriate modifications.

When following a vegetarian or vegan macro diet, it is crucial to ensure an adequate intake of protein, as it is an essential macronutrient for muscle repair, cell growth, and overall health. Vegetarian sources of protein include beans, lentils, chickpeas, tofu, tempeh, seitan, edamame, and various types of legumes. Vegans can also incorporate plant-based protein powders such as pea, rice, hemp, or soy protein to meet their protein requirements.

In terms of carbohydrates, both vegetarians and vegans have a wide range of options. Whole grains like quinoa, brown rice, oats, and whole wheat products are excellent sources of complex carbohydrates. Fruits, vegetables, and starchy vegetables like potatoes, sweet potatoes, and corn are also rich sources of carbohydrates. It's important to focus on whole, unprocessed foods to maximize nutrient intake and minimize added sugars.

For dietary fats, vegetarians can include sources like eggs, dairy products, and plant-based oils such as olive oil, avocado oil, and coconut oil. Vegans can incorporate fats from plant-based sources like avocados, nuts, seeds, and their respective oils. It is important to choose healthy fats in moderation to support overall health and meet the caloric requirements of the diet.

When adapting the macro diet for vegetarian or vegan lifestyles, it's essential to monitor and adjust macronutrient ratios based on individual needs and goals. Consulting a registered dietitian or nutritionist can provide personalized guidance to ensure adequate nutrient intake.

In addition to macronutrients, it is crucial to pay attention to micronutrients such as iron, vitamin B12, zinc, and omega-3 fatty acids, which may require special attention in vegetarian or vegan diets. Iron can be obtained from plant-based sources like legumes, dark leafy greens, and fortified cereals. Vitamin B12, primarily found in animal products, should be supplemented in vegan diets through fortified foods or supplements. Omega-3 fatty acids can be found in plant-based foods such as walnuts, hemp seeds, chia seeds, and flaxseeds. Zinc can be obtained from legumes, whole grains, nuts, and seeds.

Therefore, the following are 10 vegetarian and vegan recipes that can be incorporated into a macro diet:

1. Quinoa and Black Bean Salad:
- After cooking the quinoa as directed on the package, allow it to cool.
- In a bowl, combine cooked quinoa, black beans, diced vegetables (bell peppers, tomatoes, red onions), and chopped cilantro.
- For the dressing, whisk together lime juice, olive oil, minced garlic, cumin, salt, and pepper. Pour the salad dressing over it and toss to mix it in.

2. Tofu Stir-Fry:
- Squeeze and drain tofu, before slicing it into cubes.

- In a hot skillet, sauté diced vegetables (such as bell peppers, broccoli, and carrots) in a small amount of oil.
- Add tofu cubes and stir-fry until lightly browned and heated through.
- Season with soy sauce, ginger, garlic, and a touch of sesame oil. Serve over brown rice or quinoa.

3. Lentil and Vegetable Curry:
- Ginger, garlic, and diced onions should be sautéed in a big pot.
- Add diced vegetables (such as carrots, cauliflower, and bell peppers) and cook until slightly tender.
- Stir in cooked lentils, coconut milk, curry powder, turmeric, cumin, and salt.
- Simmer until the flavors meld together. Eat with brown rice or whole wheat naan bread.

4. Chickpea Salad Wrap:
- In a bowl, combine cooked chickpeas, diced cucumber, cherry tomatoes, red onions, chopped parsley, and a squeeze of lemon juice.
- Toss in with salt, pepper, and a tiny bit of olive oil.
- Spoon the mixture onto a whole wheat wrap or tortilla, and fold it into a wrap.

5. Vegan Protein Pancakes:
- In a mixing bowl, combine mashed bananas, plant-based protein powder, almond flour, almond milk, and a pinch of baking powder.
- Mix until well combined and let the batter rest for a few minutes.
- Cook the pancakes on a lightly oiled griddle or non-stick pan until golden brown on both sides.

- Garnish with a teaspoon of pure maple syrup and some fresh fruit.

6. Sweet Potato and Black Bean Chili:
- Sauté diced onions and minced garlic in a large pot until fragrant.
- Add diced sweet potatoes, black beans, diced tomatoes, vegetable broth, and spices like chili powder, cumin, paprika, and salt.
- Simmer for the sweet potatoes to become soft and the flavors to combine. Add some chopped cilantro on top before serving.

7. Vegan Buddha Bowl:
- Roast a variety of vegetables like Brussels sprouts, broccoli, carrots, and sweet potatoes in the oven with a drizzle of olive oil, salt, and pepper.
- Prepare brown rice or quinoa per the directions on the package.
- Assemble the bowl with the roasted vegetables, cooked grains, and add-ons like avocado slices, hummus, and a sprinkle of seeds.

8. Vegan Protein Smoothie:
- Blend together frozen berries, a scoop of vegan protein powder, almond milk, a handful of spinach or kale, and a tablespoon of nut butter.
- Adjust the consistency by adding extra liquid as needed.
- Pour into a glass and enjoy it as a post-workout or on-the-go meal.

9. Vegan Lentil Bolognese:

- Sauté diced onions, carrots, and celery in a pan until softened.
- Add cooked lentils, crushed tomatoes, tomato paste, garlic, dried herbs (such as oregano and basil), salt, and pepper.
- Let the flavors merge together by simmering for around 20 minutes. Toss with zucchini noodles or whole wheat spaghetti.

10. Vegan Protein Power Bowl:
- Cooked quinoa or brown rice is a good starting point..
- Top with a mix of protein-rich ingredients like roasted chickpeas, grilled tofu or tempeh, steamed edamame, and avocado slices.
- Add a variety of vegetables, such as steamed broccoli, shredded carrots, and sliced cucumbers.
- Drizzle with a dressing made from tahini, lemon juice, garlic, and a splash of water.

In summary, adapting the macro diet for vegetarian or vegan lifestyles involves careful consideration of protein sources, carbohydrate choices, and healthy fats. It is important to focus on a variety of whole, unprocessed foods to ensure adequate nutrient intake and to monitor micronutrient needs. Consulting a healthcare professional or registered dietitian can provide personalized guidance to optimize the diet based on individual goals and preferences.

-GLUTEN-FREE AND DAIRY-FREE OPTIONS

Following a gluten-free and dairy-free macro diet can be challenging, but with the right ingredients and recipes, it's entirely possible to create flavorful and filling meals that meet your nutritional needs. Here are some gluten-free and dairy-free options for each macronutrient category:

1. Carbohydrates:
- Quinoa: This versatile gluten-free grain is packed with protein and fiber. Use it as a basis for salads, stir-frying, or as an additional dish.
- Brown Rice: A nutrient-rich alternative to white rice, brown rice can be used in various dishes like stir-fries, grain bowls, and pilafs.
- Sweet Potatoes: These nutrient-dense tubers are a great source of carbohydrates. Enjoy them roasted, mashed, or spiralized as a noodle substitute.
- Gluten-Free Oats: Look for certified gluten-free oats to make oatmeal, granola, or use them as a flour substitute in baked goods.

2. Proteins:
- Chicken Breast: Lean and versatile, chicken breast can be grilled, baked, or sautéed for a high-protein meal.
- Turkey: Ground turkey is a lean option for making burgers, meatballs, or chili.
- Fish: Opt for gluten-free and dairy-free protein sources such as salmon, cod, or shrimp. These can be grilled, baked, or pan-seared.

- Legumes: Incorporate plant-based proteins such as lentils, chickpeas, and black beans into your meals. They can be used in salads, soups, or stews.

3. Fats:
    - Avocado: Rich in healthy fats, avocados are a great addition to salads, wraps, or enjoyed as a spread.
    - Nuts and Seeds: Flaxseeds, chia seeds, walnuts, and almonds are all great providers of heart-healthy fats. Use them in smoothies, salads, or as toppings for yogurt alternatives.
    - Coconut Milk: This creamy dairy-free alternative can be used in curries, soups, or smoothies to add richness and flavor.
    - Olive Oil: A staple in many kitchens, olive oil is ideal for sautéing vegetables or making homemade dressings and marinades.

4. Vegetables:
    - Broccoli: Rich in fiber and nutrients, broccoli can be steamed, roasted, or stir-fried as a side dish or added to main courses.
    - Spinach: Packed with nutrients, spinach can be used in salads, sautés, or added to smoothies.
    - Bell Peppers: Colorful and crunchy, bell peppers are versatile and can be used in stir-fries, salads, or stuffed with proteins.
    - Zucchini: Spiralize zucchini to create "zoodles" as a gluten-free alternative to pasta or use them in stir-fries and casseroles.

5. Snacks and Desserts:
- Fresh Fruits: Enjoy a variety of fresh fruits as snacks or blend them into smoothies.
- Rice Cakes: Gluten-free rice cakes can be topped with nut butter, avocado, or hummus for a quick snack.
- Dark Chocolate: Look for dairy-free dark chocolate options for a satisfying and antioxidant-rich treat.
- Homemade Energy Balls: Make your own energy balls using gluten-free oats, nut butters, seeds, and dried fruits.

Furthermore, the following are the lists of 10 gluten-free and dairy-free recipes that are suitable for a macro diet, along with their preparations:

1. Quinoa Salad with Roasted Vegetables:
- Cook quinoa according to package instructions.
- Roast a variety of vegetables like bell peppers, zucchini, and eggplant in the oven with olive oil, salt, and pepper.
- Toss the cooked quinoa with the roasted vegetables, fresh herbs (such as parsley or basil), lemon juice, and a drizzle of olive oil.

2. Grilled Chicken with Sweet Potato Mash:
- Grill chicken breasts seasoned with salt, pepper, and herbs.
- Boil peeled sweet potatoes until tender, then mash them with coconut milk, garlic powder, and salt.

3. Lentil Curry with Cauliflower Rice:
   - Sauté onions, minced garlic, and curry paste in a
     pot.
   - Add cooked lentils, diced tomatoes, coconut milk,
     and cauliflower rice.
   - Simmer until the flavors meld together and the
     cauliflower rice is tender.

4. Baked Salmon with Lemon and Herbs:
   - Season salmon filets with lemon zest, minced
     garlic, dried herbs, salt, and pepper.
   - Bake in the oven until the salmon is cooked to
     your liking.

5. Turkey and Vegetable Stir-Fry:
   - Sauté ground turkey, diced onions, minced garlic,
     and a mix of vegetables like bell peppers, snap peas,
     and carrots.
   - Season with gluten-free soy sauce or tamari,
     ginger, and a touch of honey or maple syrup.

6. Gluten-Free Chicken Tacos with Lettuce Wraps:
   - Marinate chicken strips in a mixture of lime juice,
     cumin, paprika, garlic powder, and salt.
   - Cook the chicken in a skillet until browned and
     cooked through.
   - Serve the chicken with lettuce leaves as wraps
     and top with salsa, avocado, and cilantro.

7. Shrimp and Vegetable Stir-Fry with Rice Noodles:
   - Sauté peeled shrimp, minced garlic, and a mix of
     vegetables like bell peppers, broccoli, and carrots.

- Cook gluten-free rice noodles according to package instructions.
- Toss the cooked noodles with the stir-fried shrimp and vegetables, and season with gluten-free soy sauce or tamari.

8. Baked Chicken Thighs with Roasted Brussels Sprouts:

- Season chicken thighs with salt, pepper, and a sprinkle of paprika.
- Arrange the chicken on a baking sheet along with halved Brussels sprouts.
- Bake until the chicken is cooked through and the Brussels sprouts are crispy.

9. Gluten-Free Beef Stir-Fry with Quinoa:

- Sauté sliced beef, diced onions, minced garlic, and a mix of vegetables like mushrooms, snow peas, and bok choy.
- Season with gluten-free soy sauce or tamari, ginger, and a touch of honey or maple syrup.
- Serve over cooked quinoa.

10. Vegetable Curry with Cauliflower Rice:

- Sauté diced onions, minced garlic, and curry paste in a pot.
- Add a mix of vegetables like cauliflower florets, carrots, and peas, along with coconut milk and vegetable broth.
- Cook until the flavors combine and the veggies are soft.
- Serve over cauliflower rice.

These recipes provide a range of flavors and ingredients that are gluten-free and dairy-free, making them suitable for a macro diet. Adjust portion sizes according to your macronutrient goals, and feel free to modify the recipes by adding or substituting ingredients based on your preferences and dietary restrictions. Enjoy these delicious and nutritious meals. Again, remember to read labels carefully as some processed gluten-free products may contain dairy or other allergens. Additionally, focus on whole, unprocessed foods whenever possible to ensure a balanced and nutritious macro diet.

CHAPTER 10:

TROUBLESHOOTING AND TIPS FOR SUCCESS

- OVERCOMING COMMON CHALLENGES IN MACRO MANAGEMENT.

Embarking on a macro diet journey can be both rewarding and challenging. While the principles of tracking macronutrients—proteins, fats, and carbohydrates—offer a structured approach to nutrition, various obstacles may arise along the way. To ensure sustained success, it's crucial to address these common challenges head-on.

1. Plateau Busting:
One prevalent challenge in macro management is encountering plateaus in progress. As the body adapts to changes in macronutrient intake, weight loss or muscle gain may stall. To overcome plateaus, it's essential to embrace flexibility. Tweak your macro ratios or total intake slightly to shock your system and reignite progress. This might involve adjusting the distribution of protein, fats, and carbs or altering the overall caloric intake. Small, intentional changes can help break through plateaus without compromising the overall structure of your macro plan.

2. Social Situations:
Another obstacle many individuals face is managing their macro intake in social settings. Events, gatherings, and dining out can challenge even the

most disciplined individuals. One strategy is to plan ahead. If possible, inquire about the menu beforehand and choose dishes that align with your macro goals. Additionally, consider eating a balanced meal before the event to reduce the temptation to overindulge. For more control, bring macro-friendly snacks to ensure you have options that align with your dietary plan. This proactive approach empowers individuals to navigate social situations without compromising their macro management.

3. Balancing Act:

Striking the right balance between macronutrients can be a delicate task. Some may find it challenging to meet their protein goals without exceeding their fat or carbohydrate limits. In such cases, diversifying protein sources becomes essential. Experiment with lean meats, plant-based proteins, and dairy to find a balance that suits your taste preferences and dietary requirements. The key is to be flexible and open to adjusting your macronutrient distribution to accommodate your body's unique needs.

4. Time Constraints:

In our fast-paced lives, time constraints often emerge as a significant hurdle. Preparing macro-friendly meals requires planning and organization, which may seem challenging amidst a busy schedule. To overcome this, consider batch cooking. Prepare larger quantities of macro-appropriate meals in advance and portion them for the week. Investing time in meal prep on a designated day can save precious minutes during hectic weekdays, ensuring that your nutrition remains on track, even when time is scarce.

5. Emotional Eating:

Emotional eating poses a substantial challenge for many individuals navigating a macro diet. Stress, boredom, or other emotional triggers can lead to unplanned deviations from your macro plan. Recognizing and addressing emotional eating is crucial. Developing alternative coping mechanisms such as mindfulness, exercise, or engaging in hobbies can redirect emotional impulses away from food. Additionally, having a support system to discuss challenges and emotions can contribute to a healthier relationship with food.

6. Dietary Restrictions:

For those with specific dietary restrictions or preferences, adhering to macro goals might seem daunting. However, the flexibility of macro tracking allows for customization. Whether following a vegetarian, vegan, gluten-free, or other specialized diet, it's possible to meet macro targets with careful planning. Utilize resources, recipes, and alternatives to ensure a diverse and satisfying diet within the constraints of your specific dietary requirements.

7. Lack of Variety:

Repetition in meals can lead to boredom, making it challenging to sustain a macro diet in the long run. Combatting monotony involves exploring diverse recipes and experimenting with different food combinations. Engage in meal prep sessions with a variety of ingredients to keep your taste buds stimulated. Not only does this approach make adhering to your macro plan more enjoyable, but it also ensures you obtain a broad spectrum of nutrients from different foods.

Successfully managing macronutrients requires a combination of strategy, adaptability, and perseverance. By addressing common challenges head-on, individuals can create a sustainable and personalized approach to macro management that aligns with their health and fitness goals. Whether breaking through plateaus, navigating social situations, or finding the right balance, proactive measures and a positive mindset are instrumental in overcoming the hurdles on the path to macro success.

- STAYING MOTIVATED AND CONSISTENT IN MACRO MANAGEMENT

Embarking on a macro diet journey requires not only a keen understanding of nutrition but also a steadfast commitment to staying motivated and consistent. The road to achieving and maintaining macro goals is often paved with challenges, but with the right mindset and strategies, individuals can foster lasting motivation and unwavering consistency.

1. Set Clear and Attainable Goals:
The foundation of motivation lies in having clear and achievable goals. Define specific targets for your

macro journey, whether it's losing a certain amount of weight, building muscle, or improving overall well-being. Break down large goals into smaller, manageable milestones. Celebrating these incremental victories provides a continuous sense of achievement, reinforcing your commitment to the macro lifestyle.

2. Visualize Success:

Visualization can be a powerful motivational tool. Envision the positive changes in your body, energy levels, and overall health. Visualizing success not only reinforces your goals but also serves as a constant reminder of the benefits of staying committed to your macro management plan.

3. Variety in Meals:

Maintaining enthusiasm for your macro diet requires keeping things interesting. Experiment with diverse recipes, ingredients, and cooking methods to add variety to your meals. A monotonous diet can lead to boredom and diminished motivation. Embrace the rich tapestry of foods available to you, ensuring both nutritional balance and a satisfying culinary experience.

4. Celebrate Small Wins:

Completing a week of consistently hitting your macro targets or resisting temptation in a challenging situation deserves acknowledgment. Rewarding yourself for these achievements reinforces positive behavior and strengthens your commitment to the macro lifestyle.

5. Track Progress:

Regularly monitor your progress to stay motivated. Utilize tracking tools or apps to log your meals, exercise, and overall well-being. Tracking provides tangible evidence of your dedication and offers insights into how your body responds to different macro compositions. Seeing positive changes over time serves as a powerful motivator, validating the effort you invest in your macro management journey.

6. Embrace Flexibility:

Maintain a flexible mindset to adapt to the evolving nature of your macro journey. Life is dynamic, and unexpected events or changes may occur. Instead of viewing deviations from your plan as setbacks, consider them opportunities to learn and adjust. Flexibility fosters resilience, preventing frustration and enhancing long-term adherence to your macro goals.

7. Find Joy in Exercise:

Incorporate enjoyable physical activities into your routine. It should be enjoyable to exercise rather than feeling like a duty. Whether it's a favorite sport, dance class, or outdoor activity, finding joy in movement enhances overall well-being and contributes to a positive mindset, reinforcing your commitment to the macro lifestyle.

8. Build a Support System:

Surround yourself with individuals who understand and support your macro management journey. Inform your loved ones and friends about your objectives, or join online groups to meet people who share your interests.. Having a support system provides encouragement during challenging times and creates a sense of accountability, reinforcing your commitment to macro success.

9. Reflect on Non-Scale Victories:

While tracking progress on the scale is valuable, don't overlook non-scale victories. Celebrate improvements in energy levels, sleep quality, mood, and overall well-being. These non-scale achievements often indicate the positive impact of your macro lifestyle on your holistic health, further motivating you to stay consistent.

10. Establish a Routine:

Consistency thrives in routine. Create a daily schedule that accommodates your macro goals, including dedicated times for meals, exercise, and self-care. A structured routine minimizes decision fatigue and provides a sense of stability, making it easier to stay committed to your macro management plan over the long term.

In the realm of macro management, staying motivated and consistent is a continuous journey rather than a destination. By setting clear goals, visualizing success, embracing variety, celebrating wins, and building a supportive environment, individuals can cultivate a sustainable and rewarding macro lifestyle. The key lies not just in achieving short-term results but in fostering a mindset and habits that promote lasting success on the macro management journey.

- FINDING SUPPORT AND ACCOUNTABILITY IN MACRO MANAGEMENT.

Embarking on a macro management journey is a significant commitment, and having a robust support system is crucial for success. Whether you're aiming for weight loss, muscle gain, or overall health improvement, finding support and accountability can make the difference between fleeting attempts and lasting lifestyle changes. Here's a comprehensive exploration of strategies to cultivate a support network and foster accountability in your macro management journey.

1. *Buddy System*:
   - Mutual Motivation:Partnering with someone who shares similar macro goals provides mutual motivation. This camaraderie transforms the journey into a shared experience, fostering encouragement and shared achievements.
   - Accountability Checks: Regularly check in with your macro buddy. Share your successes, challenges, and adjustments. This creates a sense of accountability, as you're not just answerable to yourself but also to your partner.

2. *Online Communities*:
   - Shared Experiences: Joining online forums or social media groups dedicated to macro management allows you to connect with individuals on similar journeys. Sharing experiences, challenges, and triumphs in a virtual space creates a supportive community.

- Access to Resources: Online communities are rich sources of information. Members often share recipes, macro-friendly tips, and troubleshooting strategies. This collective knowledge enhances your understanding of macro management.

3. *Professional Guidance:*
- Nutritionist or Dietitian:Seeking professional guidance from a nutritionist or dietitian provides personalized support. These experts can tailor macro recommendations based on your specific needs, health conditions, and fitness goals.
- Regular Check-ins:Schedule regular check-ins with your nutrition professional. These sessions offer a structured review of your progress, allowing for adjustments to your macro plan as needed.

4. *Fitness Classes or Groups*:
- Shared Goals: Joining fitness classes or groups with a focus on macro-based nutrition brings together individuals with shared health and fitness goals. This creates a supportive environment where macro management is woven into the fabric of the community.
- In-Person Accountability: The face-to-face interactions in a fitness class or group setting provide a tangible form of accountability. One of the most potent motivators is knowing that people are aware of your objectives.

5. *Family and Friends*:
- Educate and Involve:Share your macro journey with family and friends. Educate them about your

goals and the importance of macro management. Involving them in your journey can lead to a supportive environment at home.
- Meal Planning Together: Plan and prepare macro-friendly meals with family or friends. This not only strengthens your support network but also encourages healthier eating habits for everyone involved.

6. *Goal Sharing*:
- Public Commitment:Make your macro goals public, whether through social media, a blog, or discussions with friends and family. This public commitment adds a layer of accountability, as you become more conscious of your actions knowing that others are aware of your objectives.
- Progress Updates: Regularly update your support network on your progress. This transparency not only keeps you accountable but also allows others to celebrate your achievements and provide encouragement during challenging times.

7. *Accountability Apps*:
- Daily Check-Ins: Utilize accountability apps that prompt you to log your meals, exercise, and overall well-being. These apps often incorporate social features, allowing you to connect with friends or fellow users for shared accountability.
- Virtual Challenges: Engage in virtual challenges within these apps. Whether it's hitting daily macro targets or participating in fitness challenges, the competitive and collaborative aspects can enhance motivation and accountability.

8. ***Create a Macro Management Journal***:
- Reflective Practice: Maintain a journal documenting your macro journey. Include your goals, challenges, and strategies. Regularly reflect on your entries to gain insights into your habits, successes, and areas for improvement.
- Self-Accountability:The act of journaling fosters self-accountability. It's a tangible record of your commitment and progress, serving as a personal motivator.

9. ***Group Workshops or Seminars***:
- Shared Learning:Attend group workshops or seminars focused on macro management. Engaging in collective learning experiences not only expands your knowledge but also connects you with individuals who are invested in similar health goals.
- Networking Opportunities:Take advantage of networking opportunities during these events. Form connections with attendees, creating a network of individuals who can provide support and accountability.

10. ***Online Challenges:***
- Community Engagement:Participate in online challenges related to macro management. These challenges often involve a community of participants working towards similar goals. The shared experience fosters camaraderie and accountability.
- Structured Guidelines:Online challenges usually come with structured guidelines, providing a framework for your macro journey. This structure can

be particularly beneficial for those who thrive on clear goals and timelines.

However, finding support and accountability in macro management is a dynamic process that involves leveraging various resources. Whether through partnerships, online communities, professional guidance, or personal reflection, creating a robust support network significantly enhances the likelihood of success on your macro journey. Remember that accountability is not just a means to an end; it's a continuous, reciprocal relationship that fuels motivation and sustains long-term commitment to your macro management goals.

- TRACKING PROGRESS AND MAKING ADJUSTMENTS IN MACRO MANAGEMENT.

A successful macro management journey involves not just setting initial goals but also implementing a dynamic system for tracking progress and making necessary adjustments along the way. Whether your focus is on weight loss, muscle gain, or overall well-being, a meticulous approach to monitoring and adapting your macro plan is crucial for sustained success. Here's a comprehensive exploration of strategies to effectively track your progress and make informed adjustments in your macro management journey.

1. *Use Tracking Apps:*
   - Meal Logging:Invest in reputable tracking apps like MyFitnessPal to log your daily meals. These apps

offer a comprehensive database of foods, making it easier to track your macro intake accurately.
- Nutrient Breakdowns: Tracking apps provide detailed nutrient breakdowns, allowing you to assess your protein, fat, and carbohydrate consumption. Regularly review these breakdowns to ensure you're aligning with your macro targets.

2. *Regular Assessments:*
- Scheduled Check-Ins: Establish a routine for regular assessments. This could involve weekly or monthly check-ins where you evaluate your progress, assess adherence to your macro plan, and identify areas for improvement.
- Goal Reevaluation:During assessments, revisit your initial goals. Are they still realistic and relevant? Adjust them if necessary based on your evolving understanding of your body and your macro management journey.

3. *Monitor Physical Changes*:
- Body Measurements: Beyond the scale, track physical changes through body measurements. Regularly measure key areas such as waist, hips, and chest to capture a more comprehensive picture of your body's transformation.
- Progress Photos: Take progress photos at consistent intervals. Visual evidence of changes can be a powerful motivator and provides a tangible record of your macro journey.

4. *Energy Levels and Performance:*
   - Subjective Assessments: Pay attention to your energy levels and overall performance. An increase in energy and improved performance during workouts can be indicative of effective macro management.
   - Adjustment Indicators: If you experience fatigue or a decline in performance, consider whether adjustments to your macro ratios or overall intake are needed. Your body's response is valuable feedback in refining your approach.

5. *Biofeedback Signals:*
   - Hunger and Satisfaction: Listen to your body's hunger and satisfaction signals. Feeling overly hungry or consistently unsatisfied may indicate a need for adjustments in your macro distribution or total caloric intake.
   - Digestive Health: Monitor your digestive health. Unusual discomfort or digestive issues could be a signal that your body is reacting to specific macros, prompting the need for modifications.

6. *Macro Cycling:*
   - Periodic Variations: Consider incorporating macro cycling into your plan. This involves varying your macro ratios on different days to accommodate training intensity, rest days, or specific goals. Macro cycling adds flexibility and responsiveness to your nutritional approach.
   - Assess Impact: Regularly assess the impact of macro cycling on your progress. Evaluate whether it enhances your performance, supports recovery, and contributes to your overall macro management goals.

7. *Feedback Loops:*

- Solicit Feedback: Actively seek feedback from trusted sources. This could be a nutritionist, fitness coach, or individuals with expertise in macro management. External perspectives can provide valuable insights and identify blind spots in your approach.

- introspective Practices: Make introspective exercises a regular part of your day.. Regularly assess your experiences, challenges, and successes. This self-reflection enhances your understanding of your macro journey and guides adjustments.

8. *Mindful Eating:*

- Conscious Consumption:Practice mindful eating to enhance awareness of your food choices. Be present during meals, savor each bite, and pay attention to your body's signals of hunger and fullness.

- Adjust Based on Feedback:Mindful eating can reveal patterns in your dietary habits. Adjust your macros based on these patterns, ensuring that your nutritional choices align with your macro management goals.

9. *Reassess Macro Ratios:*

- Periodic Reevaluation:Macro requirements can evolve over time. Periodically reassess your macro ratios to ensure they align with your current goals, lifestyle, and body composition.

- Experimentation: Don't hesitate to experiment with different macro distributions. Your body's response to adjustments provides valuable information for fine-tuning your approach.

10. ***Consultation with Professionals:***
- Nutritional Guidance: Seek professional guidance when needed. A nutritionist or dietitian can provide personalized advice based on your individual needs, helping you navigate challenges and make informed adjustments.
- Health Check-Ups: Regular health check-ups can identify any underlying issues affecting your progress. Consult with healthcare professionals to ensure that your macro management plan aligns with your overall well-being.

Therefore, the journey of macro management is not a static path but a dynamic process that requires continuous monitoring and adjustments. Utilize tracking apps, regularly assess your progress, monitor physical changes, listen to biofeedback signals, and remain open to adjustments based on your evolving understanding of your body and goals. By embracing a flexible and proactive approach to tracking and adjusting, you empower yourself to navigate the intricacies of macro management with precision and purpose. Remember, the key to sustained success lies not only in setting goals but in the ongoing refinement of your macro management strategy.

CONCLUSION

Achieving optimal health and fitness is a multifaceted journey that encompasses dietary choices, lifestyle adjustments, and a commitment to understanding the nuanced interplay between nutrition and well-being. In delving into "The Macro Diet Cookbook for Beginners 2024," we find not just a collection of recipes but a holistic guide that equips individuals with the knowledge and tools necessary to embark on a transformative health and fitness adventure.

The overarching theme of this cookbook lies in its commitment to demystifying the macro diet—a dietary approach centered around the strategic consumption of macronutrients: proteins, fats, and carbohydrates. As we explore this culinary compendium, it becomes evident that it transcends the boundaries of a typical cookbook. It stands as an educational cornerstone, empowering readers to make informed decisions about their dietary habits, thereby facilitating lasting improvements in their health.

One of the cookbook's most commendable features is its unwavering dedication to inclusivity. Recognizing that the path to health and fitness is unique for each individual, the cookbook provides a diverse array of recipes tailored to beginners. From quick and easy meals for those with busy schedules to more elaborate dishes for those who relish spending time in the kitchen, the cookbook accommodates a spectrum of preferences and lifestyles.

Central to the cookbook's success is its commitment to education. Rather than presenting a mere list of recipes, it takes the time to elucidate the fundamental principles of the macro diet. Readers are guided through the significance of each macronutrient, the role it plays in the body, and how a balanced consumption of proteins, fats, and carbohydrates can contribute to overall well-being. This educational component transforms the cookbook into a comprehensive manual for sustainable health rather than a mere compilation of recipes.

The recipes themselves, meticulously crafted and tested, serve as a testament to the cookbook's commitment to flavor and nutrition. From breakfast options that kickstart the day with energy to satisfying dinners that fuel post-workout recovery, each recipe is a culinary exploration that marries taste and health. The incorporation of a wide variety of ingredients ensures that the macro diet doesn't become a monotonous journey but rather an exciting culinary adventure.

Beyond the kitchen, the cookbook delves into the psychological and behavioral aspects of adopting a macro-based approach to eating. It acknowledges the challenges individuals may face when transitioning to a new dietary regimen and provides practical tips for overcoming hurdles. This psychological support is integral, recognizing that a positive mindset is as crucial as the nutritional content of the meals consumed.

The cookbook's emphasis on practicality is further evident in its attention to meal planning and preparation. It recognizes the modern lifestyle's demands and offers insights into efficient planning, grocery shopping, and batch cooking. This not only streamlines the process of adhering to the macro diet but also dispels the notion that maintaining a healthy diet requires an excessive amount of time and effort.

As we reflect on the cookbook's content, it becomes apparent that it goes beyond the confines of nutrition and extends into the realms of overall wellness. It champions the notion that achieving health and fitness goals is not solely about restrictive diets but about cultivating a balanced and sustainable lifestyle. By intertwining nutritional guidance with practical tips and flavorful recipes, it facilitates a seamless integration of the macro diet into daily life.

Furthermore, the cookbook's adaptability to individual needs is a commendable aspect. Whether one's fitness goal is weight loss, muscle gain, or simply maintaining a healthy lifestyle, the cookbook offers tailored recipes and insights. This adaptability fosters a sense of agency and personalization, crucial elements in sustaining long-term commitment to health and fitness.

In a world where fad diets often dominate the conversation, "The Macro Diet Cookbook for Beginners 2024" emerges as a beacon of evidence-based guidance. It not only acknowledges the importance of macronutrients but also underscores the significance of enjoying the journey. The inclusion of diverse recipes ensures that individuals with various dietary preferences find a place within the macro framework, promoting a sense of inclusivity and accessibility.

Therefore, this cookbook transcends its title as a mere recipe collection. It stands as a comprehensive guide, a roadmap for those embarking on the journey to improved health and fitness. By demystifying the macro diet, offering a diverse array of recipes, and providing educational insights, it becomes a companion—a reliable source of support and information on the quest for a healthier and more vibrant life. As we close the pages of this culinary adventure, we emerge not just with a repertoire of delicious meals but with a newfound understanding of the intricate dance between nutrition and well-being.

www.ingramcontent.com/pod-product-compliance
Lightning Source LLC
Chambersburg PA
CBHW070900260726
48661CB00004B/1511